Derek Langford

I0414764

Intuitive Eating 2.0: Lose weight naturally and permanently, free Yourself from a Lifetime of Dieting, build a healthy relationship with food and Honor Your Feelings Without Using Food

3

Contents

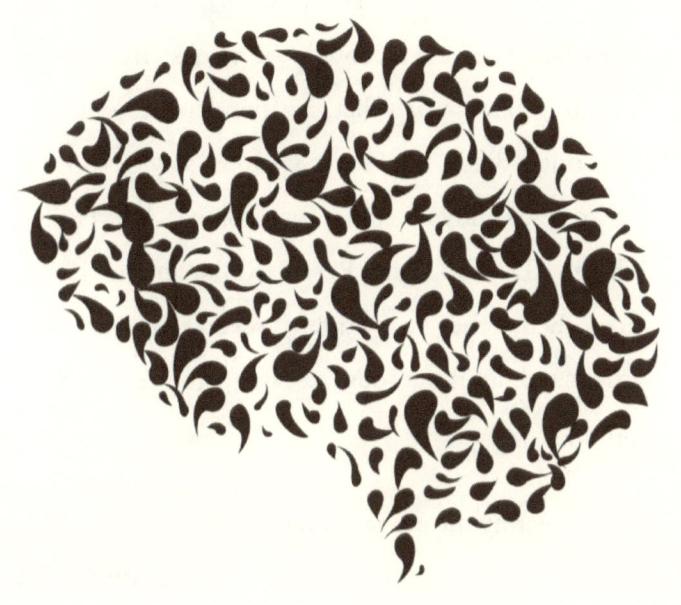

INTRODUCTION

What Is Intuitive Eating?

In this day and age, it seems like a trendy, new diet makes headlines every couple of weeks. But there's one eating plan—*not* a diet, its founders are quick to point out—that's had some serious staying power. The term intuitive eating was coined by Evelyn Tribole, RD, and Elyse Resch, RDN, in the 1990s; since then, they've written several books and participated in numerous research studies on their method.

Intuitive eating means breaking free from the on-and-off cycle of dieting and learning to eat mindfully and without guilt. There's no calorie counting but there are some guidelines—10 principles, to be exact—that make up the core philosophy of this method.

1. Reject the diet mentality

Tribole says she and Resch wrote their first book on intuitive eating after watching their patients constantly struggle with dieting. "We were sick of the insanity they were going through: They'd restrict themselves and lose weight, but then they'd gain it back and they'd blame themselves," she says. "These were intelligent, successful people, and so we really took a deep dive into the research to figure out what was going wrong."

The bottom line, Tribole says, is that dieting isn't sustainable. So the first principle of intuitive eating is to stop dieting—and to stop believing society's messages that quick-fix plans can deliver lasting results. That includes throwing away diet books and magazine articles that promise fast weight loss, and rejecting any meal plans that dictate what or how much you can eat.

2. Honor your hunger

One reason dieting doesn't work, Tribole says, is because it can leave you feeling deprived and physically hungry—which can trigger binging and overeating. So instead of counting calories or watching portions, she says, simply pay attention to your body's hunger cues.

That means eating a sufficient amount of calories and carbohydrates to keep your body "fed" and satiated. Once you learn to recognize these signals in your own body, Tribole says, it becomes much easier to trust your instincts and repair unhealthy relationships with food.

3. Make peace with food

"When you're on a diet, certain foods are promoted as being forbidden—which tends to make them even more tempting," says Tribole. "Then when you finally eat those foods, you binge and feel guilty, which creates a vicious cycle." That's why one principle of intuitive eating is to give yourself "unconditional permission to eat." It may sound like a recipe for all-out gluttony, but Tribole says it almost never plays out that way.

"A wonderful thing ends up happening when you give yourself permission to, say, eat chocolate doughnuts for breakfast," she says. "You stop and ask yourself, 'Do I really want this now?' Not just, 'Will I enjoy it in the moment,' but also 'Will I feel good when I'm finished?' And often, people realize they don't really want that food that was forbidden before; they just got caught up in society telling them they couldn't have it."

4. Challenge the food police

Intuitive eating describes the "food police" as those voices in your head that tell you it's good to eat fewer calories and it's bad to eat dessert; in other words, it's your psyche's way of monitoring all of the dieting rules you've heard again and again over the years and making you feel guilty for not following them to the letter.

These food police can be real people, too, says Tribole: friends, family, and acquaintances who offer up judgment and "advice" about what and how you're eating. In either case, she says, "chasing them away" is an important step in embracing intuitive eating.

5. Respect your fullness

This goes hand-in-hand with principle #2. Yes, it's important to eat when you're hungry, but it's also important to stop when those hunger cues are no longer present.

It can help to pause in the middle of your meal or snack to assess your current state: How full do you feel? Are you still eating to feed your hunger, or are you eating out of distraction, boredom, or stress? "We all have the power to listen to our bodies in this way, but many people don't realize it," says Tribole.

6. Discover the satisfaction factor

The satisfaction factor has to do with noticing and appreciating the taste and texture of food, but also the environment in which you're eating. "This is the hub of intuitive eating," says Tribole. "If we start here and aim for satisfaction, everything else falls into place."

Getting satisfaction from your food is about truly understanding what feels good and what doesn't. "Most people have never asked themselves the question, 'What do I like to eat? What feels good in my body?'" Tribole says. "When you can bring the pleasure and joy back to eating, you can truly feel satisfied after a meal and move on and enjoy the rest of your life, rather than continue to eat for other reasons."

To put this into practice, Tribole recommends starting with just one meal a day. "Make it a sacred time in which you eat without distraction," she says. "Place your awareness on one aspect of the food, whether it's the texture or the taste or the visual aspect." If even that sounds too difficult to do with your busy schedule, concentrate on just the first bite, the middle bite, and the last bite.

7. Honor your feelings without using food

Speaking of "other reasons," Tribole says that people often overeat because of anxiety, loneliness, boredom, anger, or stress. That's why it's important to get to the root of these problems, and to find ways to nurture yourself and resolve those issues without turning to food.

"It's not always big, extreme emotions that are causing overeating, either," says Tribole. "Sometimes it's as mundane as being bored because you're eating while distracted." But being more mindful in all aspects of life—with your food and with your emotions—can help you sort out those overlaps.

8. Respect your body

Intuitive eating is also about body acceptance: That means feeling good about your "genetic blueprint" and the body you were meant to have—not striving for unrealistic expectations about how much weight you can lose or what size jeans you can squeeze into.

It's also important to understand that intuitive eating is not a weight-loss plan, although Tribole says that some women do lose weight (and keep it off) once they leave behind their unhealthy history with dieting and food restriction.

9. Exercise: Feel the difference

You don't have to go to the gym every day while following an intuitive eating approach, but it is important to move your body on a regular basis. "It's not about finding the exercise that burns the most calories or the most fat," says Tribole. "It's about finding something that's sustainable and that you enjoy."

Exercise has many benefits that even the healthiest eating plan can't convey on its own, Tribole adds: It's been shown to boost mood, strengthen the heart and cardiovascular system, and increase lean muscle mass, to name a few—all things that can help you feel comfortable and powerful in your own skin.

10. Honor your health with gentle nutrition

Despite the fact that intuitive eating preaches an "eat what you want" mentality, that doesn't mean its founders don't care about good nutrition. In fact, their final word of advice is to make food choices that honor your health, as well as your taste buds.

"This last principle is probably the least controversial one, so it doesn't get talked about as much," says Tribole. "We're not throwing the baby out with the bathwater: We still encourage healthy eating, but we know that comes naturally when you embrace the other principles first."

In other words, eating "intuitively" should still involve more fruits and veggies than ice cream. But at the same time, a diet doesn't have to be perfect to be healthy, and you shouldn't beat yourself up every time you make a less-than-perfect meal or snack choice.

Health's nutritionist weighs in

So can intuitive eating really help people establish a healthy relationship with food and with their bodies—and is it really okay to kiss dieting goodbye, once and for all? Tribole says yes.

"One of the biggest misconceptions is that, without a structured diet, people will start to be unhealthy," she says. "But if you look at the research, it's clear that intuitive eaters have higher self-esteem, higher well-being, and they also tend to have lower body mass indexes. They eat a variety of foods, they have more trust in their bodies—it's really rather lovely all of the good that comes out of this."

Sass agrees that there are a lot of great things about intuitive eating, and she incorporates many of these principles into her recommendations to clients. But she also thinks that some additional structure isn't a bad thing.

"In my experience, intuitive eating can free someone from a dieting mentality that has kept someone stuck in a vicious good/bad cycle—and breaking that pattern is a very good thing," she says. "But I have also seen intuitive eating lead to imbalanced eating and confusion about what really does feel balanced."

Yes, it's true that humans are born with an instinctive sense of balance, which is why babies eat when they're hungry and stop when they're full. "But as adults, we're faced with a number of social and emotional eating triggers on a daily basis," Sass points out. And today more than ever, it can be difficult to tease out which messages are coming from our bodies versus our brains or outside sources like peer pressure or the media.

So, Why Intuitive Eating 2.0?

How to transform "Intuitive Eating" in a Intuitive nutritional therapy?

Basically, a Intuitive nutritional therapy is selecting foods that are clean, natural and nourishing. Wholesome, beneficial, healthful. Clean means to wash it, and handle it properly so that it is not contaminated, after you purchase. But, more so, it is important that the foods we eat have no chemicals added that are known to be harmful. (Believe it or not packaged and processed foods have more chemicals and additives than you can even imagine. You would think that living in this country, our food would be free of harmful additives. Think again, then read the ingredients labels. The foods we select to eat for a Intuitive nutritional therapy should be locally grown. Foods imported from far away lose a lot of the important nutrients in transport, are often sprayed with preservatives, and are irradiated to be accepted into this country. Foods should be as natural as when they came from the earth, at the time we eat them. So when you look at that package of instant mashed potatoes, you know it did not grow in the box. Organic foods, because of the way they are grown, contain more nutrients than conventionally grown foods in this country. It is because of the many poisonous chemical treatments; herbicides, pesticides, hormones and other actions the plants are subjected to that make our food supply inherently less nutritious. (However, if you continue to purchase these foods special handling is required.) Soak, rinse, or scrub fruits and vegetables before cooking and eating. Always. So, this is the condensed version of how to eat: Cook at home. Cook, prepare your own foods, and take your lunch, it will be 'cleaner', healthier and you will have more peace of mind about it.

- Eat lots of fruits and veggies.

- Have at least 2 vegetarian meals per week, more is better.

- Eat only the lean meat and poultry. (That means no wings).

- Select only 100% whole grains. Pasta, rice, bread,

whatever.

- Try to eat at least 8 servings of fruits and veggies each day. (having a salad and veggies twice a day will make this tip a snap.

- Use extra virgin olive oil on salad, toasted whole wheat bread, or in pesto on pasta. This is a great way to get the 'good fats' into your diet.

- Eat more fish. Salmon, mackerel, sardines, herrings and trout. Always choose wild caught.

You are what you eat, so if you are eating chips, sodas, burgers, chicken, and pizza from the drive through, mashed potatoes from a box, peas and corn from the can, and cereal or sausage biscuits for breakfast, you are 'doing it' all wrong. Doing it wrong sets you up for all kinds of illness and disease, and the inability to fight disease and recover well from an episode. It is true, you are what you eat. Eating a Intuitive nutritional therapy, grows a healthy person. A person with normal blood sugar, normal cholesterol, no heart disease. Illness is so common in our society that most people think it is normal to have drugs and doctors for these now common ailments. The right diet can prevent, and reverse disease.

Eliminate from your menu all processed meats. - ham, salami, hot dogs, bacon and all smoked or cured meats. These all contain nitrates and are linked to stomach and pancreatic cancer. Drink lots of water. One half your bodys' weight, in ounces of water, every day. Water is the easiest and fastest way to detox. And that is important. We make our own toxins, and water helps to eliminate them, fast. Reduce artificial preservatives, colorings, flavorings and artificial sweeteners. Avoid white sugar, especially if you are already suffering with some illness. Sugar only makes it worse. Stay away from cakes, cookies, candy, desserts, and soda, (and anything else made with white sugar). Lastly, don't feed your allergies. If you are allergic to any food, don't eat it. Common food allergies include wheat, eggs, nuts, milk, soy, and shellfish. Persons can develop an allergy to any food. So, if you don't feel good when you eat certain foods, take it off the menu.

So, look at your diet, and see how you can make it better. And do it, because you are worth it.

CHAPTER ONE

Natural food is basically the food that can be found in nature and consumed in its original form without baking it. For centuries people have known that these foods are beneficial for a healthy living. The scientific reason for this however is not known to many. Furthermore, with the spoilt food habits of children nowadays who prefer to consume junk food than natural foods, it is essential that this reason is known to them but then education is not enough. From my observation, parents should lead the correct example at home.

Unnatural foods that are consumed by us produce toxins in the body that leads to various diseases. However, these toxins can further be destroyed by an increased consumption of natural foods thereby eradicating and making an individual free from almost or at least minimize all diseases that he would suffer from. Some of the doctors even claim that the natural foods even have the power for the growth of new hair and teeth in people in their old age. Not forgetting that medical bills can wipe out all your savings overnight! Additionally, the cooling effect and their nutrients of the natural and juicy fruits such as watermelon, orange and many others that are found in summers are known to all of us. Similarly, there are other seasonal fruits and vegetables that provide high nutritional value.

People these days worry more about satisfying their taste buds rather than the nutritional requirements of their body. Most of us eat vegetables and fruits that have been peeled and in the process we also peel off the fiber, minerals and vitamins that are contained in them. Several naturopaths are of the opinion that natural products are present in their holistic form and thereby the effect that it has is also holistic, which is destroyed when the food is cooked. Millions of people are committing slow suicide with their unhealthy, inactive lifestyle, heavy consumption of meat, high sugar and high fat diets. Not to mention heavy smoking, alcohol consumption and drugs. All these things damage their organs and the inside of their arteries. Thus, adding more health issues to themselves and problems to the lives of their loved ones. Once we realize the harm caused to our body by unhealthy refined, chemical saturated, deficient foods, we'll want to eliminate these killer food. Reduce when possible all microwave food. Follow these guidelines to provide the basic healthy nourishment to maintain wellness and lifestyle:

Reduce refined sugar and artificial sweeteners: That can be found in jams, jellies, yogurt, ice cream, sherbet, jello, cake candy, cookies, chewing gums, soft drinks, pies, pastries, puddings.

Reduce white flour products such as white bread, enriched flours, rye bread, dumplings, biscuits, buns, gravy, pasta, pancakes, waffles, soda crackers, pizza, ravioli, pies, pastries, cakes, cookies send ready mix bakery products. (Insist on 100% whole grain products.)

Reduce salted food such as corn chips, potato chips, pretzels, crackers and nuts.

Reduce fried and greasy food and refined white rice.

Reduce food that contains palm and cottonseed oil.

(Not recommended for human consumption).

Peanuts and peanut butter that contains hydrogenated, hardened oil and any mold that can cause allergies.

Reduce Margarine - full of dangerous, unnatural, trans-fatty acids. (It's a no no).

Reduce saturated fat and hydrogenated oils - enemies that clog the arteries.

Reduce coffee, decaffeinated coffee, China black tea and all alcohol beverages.

Reduce pork and pork products especially fried and greasy meats.

Reduce smoked meat such as ham, bacon, sausage, bologna, corned beef, pastrami and packaged meat containing dangerous sodium nitrate or nitrite.

Reduce dried fruit containing sulphur dioxide - a toxic preservative.

Reduce consuming chicken or turkey that have been injected with hormones or fed with any drugs or toxins.

Read labels on canned soups for sugar, starch, flour and preservative concentration.

Reduce day-old cooked vegetables, potatoes and premixed wilted salads.

Reduce all commercial vinegar especially pasteurized, filtered, distilled, white, malt and synthetic.

Enjoy eating and protecting our health with Natural Food:

1. Raw food: Use fruits and raw vegetables especially organically grown. Enjoy nutritious variety garden salads with sprouts and raw nuts and seeds.

2. Vegetable and Animal Proteins:

a. Lentils, brown rice, soy beans or beans.

b. Nuts and seeds, raw and unsalted.

c.Animal protein - hormone free meats, liver, kidney, brain, heart, poultry and seafood. (Note: Please eat these proteins sparingly or it's best to enjoy the healthier vegetarian diet. It is best to bake, roast, Wok or broil these proteins. It is good idea to consume meat no more than 3 times a week).

d.Dairy Products - eggs, unprocessed hard cheese, goat cheese and certified raw milk. Try instead healthier soy, nut and Rice Dream non-dairy milks.

3. Fruits and Vegetables: Organically grown is always the best. (Grown with poisonous sprays and toxic chemical fertilizers are dangerous) Steam, bake, saute`, or Wok veggies for a short time as possible to retain the best nutritional content and flavor. Always enjoy fresh juices.

4. 100% whole grain cereals, breads and flours: They contain the most important B-complex vitamins, vitamin E, minerals and unsaturated fatty acids.

5. Cold vegetable oils: Extra Virgin Olive oil, soy, sunflower, flax and sesame oil are excellent sources of healthy, essential, unsaturated fatty acids. It's good idea to use oil consumption sparingly. And avoid dip frying.

Natural Foods to Control Blood Pressure

Generally people tend to eat processed foods like chips, or cookies when they feel hungry. This is not a healthy habit as these foods tend to increase hypertension. It is better to keep healthy low calorie foods in reach to eat whenever you feel hungry. There are several natural foods that control hypertension.

Fruits

Fruits are rich in nutrients. They are ideal snacks to lower blood pressure. Fruits are an essential ingredient of a Intuitive nutritional therapy. They contain anti-oxidants and vitamins. They can be consumed raw or in the form of salads and juices. Some of the fruits that help to manage hypertension are prunes, melons, banana and citrus fruits.

Prunes are sweet to taste and contain and high quantity of potassium. Potassium helps to maintain the blood pressure and cardiac function. They are also helpful in the prevention of atherosclerosis.

Bananas are also rich in potassium and contain very low quantities of sodium. Two bananas a day are recommended to keep the blood pressure under check.

Melons contain potassium and magnesium. They also contain carotenoids which help to prevent the hardening and narrowing of the arteries. This largely contributes to the lowering the blood pressure. Both watermelon and muskmelon have these properties.

Citrus fruits are rich in vitamin C. They also contain phytonutrients and bioflavonoids which are anti inflammatory and help to prevent blood clots. They help to control cholesterol and hypertension. Some of the important citrus fruits are orange, lime, lemon and grapefruit.

Vegetables

Vegetables help to regulate and control blood pressure. Eating more vegetables and lowering the sodium intake is essential to control blood pressure. Vegetables can be consumed raw, cooked or boiled.

Garlic is a very important vegetable that can help control hypertension. Cut three cloves of garlic into pieces and swallow it as you swallow tablets every day. This definitely is a great help in controlling hypertension. The swallowing is meant to reduce the pungent odor of garlic from the mouth.

Onion can help control blood pressure. Eating raw onion is helpful in controlling hypertension but also fight atherosclerosis, bronchitis. It helps to control irregular heart beat. Onion contains an antibiotic called allicin which is destroyed when it is cooked. Carrots, broccoli, and tomatoes are also quite useful in controlling hypertension.

CHAPTER TWO

Bring Health to Your Table With a Bounty of Natural Foods

An important reason why many people are struggling with weight or health issues is that the foods we tend to consume are largely processed, refined, and loaded with unhealthy oils, chemicals, and additives. While changing your diet isn't easy, the true path to lasting wellness involves replacing processed foods with natural foods. By giving your body a break from the constant stress involved in detoxing, digesting, and eliminating processed foods, you can truly alter the state of your body and mind and replenish yourself with healthy choices. A balanced diet is the best way to get the nutrition that you need on a daily basis. A solid diet will give your more vitality and energy and it will help you stay at your proper weight. It will also help boost your immune system and can actually help to reduce the signs of aging. What are considered natural foods? Anything that doesn't have to be canned, cooked, processed, or chemically altered in order for you to eat it: organic fruits and vegetables, nuts and seeds, and whole grains, to name a few.

While the raw food movement touts eating absolutely no cooked foods as the way to lasting health, choosing whole foods that are only lightly cooked is a great alternative to giving up your favorite dishes. By lightly cooking your meals, important enzymes in the food remain in tact that literally help your body digest it. The natural enzymes in processed foods or foods cooked at high temperatures are killed off by the heat, rendering them much more difficult for your body to break down. Taking the extra time to plan meals with natural, whole foods will immensely help on your path to holistic health and wellness. As the old adage goes, we are what we eat, so it makes sense that we should care for our bodies by giving it the nourishment needed to maintain a high metabolism, fight off disease, and function at optimal performance in our daily activities. Often, half the battle in changing our eating habits is knowing where to start, what to buy, and how to develop a plan for healthy meals and snacking. To truly give yourself an advantage, consult a holistic nutrition expert who can help you develop a strategy based on your own personal needs and goals.

Nutritional Elements of Food and Healthy Eating

The purpose of consuming food is to ensure good health and wellness, and therefore, healthy eating is an essential aspect of eating every day. The requirement of food over the years changes over time, with respect to the stage of life that you are in. So while a child requires food to grow and develop, adults need it more for the energy required to function daily. In addition to that, food is also required so as to repair the various parts of the body that are worn away, or those that have had to be discarded due to wear and tear. We tend to use various parts of our bodies with everything that we do, be it breathing, thinking, moving, playing or working on the computer. This means that we need to be able to continuously replenish our body with a variety of elements that are present in food and drink.

The various elements of food that exist, their characteristics, the manner in which they can be used, and the right way in which specific foods should be combined to obtain maximum benefits are given below:

The Food Elements

Healthy eating is possible only when you ensure that your body is getting the right food elements in the right quantity that it requires. Therefore, it is essential to know about the food nutrition to be able to make sure that you are consuming everything. Some of the food elements that you should be aware of include starch, sugar, albumen, fats, minerals, and indigestible ingredients.

These are often clubbed together to form the basic classes including carbonaceous, nitrogenous, and inorganic. While all the starches, fats and sugars fall under the carbonaceous category, the albumen is considered to be nitrogenous. All inorganic substances include all the minerals that we need for the body. It should be noted that all healthy recipes or menus should ensure that all the various categories of food are finely balanced in a meal.

Carbonaceous - All starches, sugars and fats are covered under this category. Starch can be found in grains, most vegetables, and also in some fruits. Sugars are available in the form of cane, grape, other fruit sugars, and milk sugar (a constituent of milk).There are also some sugars that are made in the laboratory.

Glucose, for example, is an artificial sugar that is similar to grape juice. It is made from potato or corn starch in a chemical process. However, it is not as sweet as the natural sweeteners that nature provides. Fats can be found in vegetables and animal food too. Butter and suet are examples of animal fat, but you can also find fat in plant sources like nuts, beans and some fruits like olives too.

While fat is commonly used as a free element (as in butter) and we use it in many not-so-healthy recipes in abundance, not only is free fat difficult to consume, but it also interferes with the digestion of other foods.

Nitrogenous - Albumen in its purest form can be found in the white of an egg. The entire white of an egg is nothing but pure albumen. You can also find albumen in other animals and vegetable foods as in the case of oatmeal. Gluten closely resembles albumen and is also a nitrogenous element. It is found in rye, barley and wheat. Casein is also a part of this class of food elements and can be found in peas and beans.

Inorganic - Almost all the foods we consume have a certain proportion of inorganic and mineral matter. Grains and milk have a large proportion of the minerals that we need on a daily basis.

Indigestible substances - These are foods that are not digestible by the body and are therefore only meant to provide bulk to the food that we eat. Bran and fibrous tissues in the body are examples of indigestible foods.

Food Element Uses

Most of the food that we eat is carbonaceous in nature. This is something that has been proven after studying the daily eating habits of various cultures. The carbonaceous food element allows our body to produce heat, and in conjunction with other food elements, allows us to be able to use force and strength. Carbonaceous food elements also help the body replace the fatty tissue that gets used up in the process of fat burning.

While fats produce the highest amount of heat among the carbonaceous food elements, it should be remembered that these are most difficult to digest and can therefore lead to various health issues. Healthy eating deems that only the recommended proportion of fat should be included in meals on a daily basis.

The nitrogenous nutritional elements help in keeping the brain, nerves, and muscles healthy and fit. These are the food elements that ensure that you remain healthy in all respects including mental health. All healthy recipes should include a decent proportion of nitrogenous food elements to ensure that the stimulus to tissue change is provided to the body at all times, thus keeping all tissues fighting fit.

The most commonly required inorganic elements are phosphates. These provide the building blocks for bones and nerves and are therefore critical for good bone health.

Combination of Food Elements

There is a saying that 'too much of everything is bad', and this applies to food as well. While all food elements are required by the body, it is necessary that each of the food elements be consumed in a specific proportion to ensure healthy eating and healthy living. If you want to learn how to cook healthy recipes, you need to know which of the food elements are required by the body and in what quantity.

Reasons to Eat Real Food

Real food is whole, single-ingredient food. It is mostly unprocessed, free of chemical additives and rich in nutrients. In essence, it's the type of food human beings ate exclusively for thousands of years. However, ever since ready-to-eat foods became popular in the 20th century, many people have been eating them as a dominant part of their diet. While processed foods may be more convenient in some ways, it's hard to argue that they have made us healthier or happier. In fact, following a diet based on real food may be one of the most important things you can do to maintain good health and high quality of life. Here are 21 reasons to eat real food.

1. Real Food Is Loaded With Important Nutrients

Unprocessed animal and plant foods contain the vitamins and minerals you need for optimal health. For instance, one cup (220 grams) of red bell peppers, broccoli or orange slices contains more than 100% of the RDI for vitamin C. Eggs and liver are especially high in choline, a nutrient that's essential for proper brain function And just a single Brazil nut provides all the selenium you need for an entire day. There are many other examples of this. In fact, most real foods are good sources of vitamins, minerals and other beneficial nutrients. Unlike supplements, it's nearly impossible to overdose on most nutrients from unprocessed food.

2. Real Food Is Low in Sugar

Some research suggests that eating sugary foods can increase your risk of obesity, insulin resistance, type 2 diabetes, fatty liver disease and heart disease.Generally speaking, real food is low in sugar and isn't very sweet. Even though fruit contains sugar, it's also high in water and fiber, so it's much less concentrated than sugar in soda and processed foods.

3. Real Food Is Heart-Healthy

Real food is packed with antioxidants and nutrients that support heart health, including magnesium and healthy fats. Eating a diet rich in nutritious, unprocessed foods may also help reduce inflammation, which is believed to be one of the major drivers of heart disease.

4. Real Food Is Good for the Environment

The world population is steadily growing, and with this growth comes increased demand for food. However, producing food to feed several billion people is taking a huge toll on the environment. This is mainly due to increased fuel needs, greenhouse gases and packaging that ends up in landfills.

On the other hand, developing sustainable systems based on real food may help improve the health of our planet by reducing energy needs and decreasing the amount of non-biodegradable waste humans produce

5. Real Food Is High in Fiber

Fiber provides many health benefits. These include helping you feel more satisfied with fewer calories, as well as improving digestive function and metabolic health. Foods such as avocados, chia seeds, flaxseeds and blackberries are particularly high in healthy fiber, along with beans and legumes. Getting fiber as it naturally occurs in real food is much better than taking a fiber supplement or eating processed food with added fiber.

6. Real Food Helps Control Blood Sugar

According to the International Diabetes Federation, more than 400 million people have diabetes worldwide. That number is expected to surpass 600 million within the next 25 years. Eating a diet high in fibrous plants and unprocessed animal foods may help reduce blood sugar levels in people with diabetes and people who are at risk of developing the disease. In one 12-week study, people with diabetes or prediabetes followed a paleolithic diet containing fresh meat, fish, fruits, vegetables, eggs and nuts. They experienced a 26% reduction in blood sugar levels.

7. Real Food Is Good for Your Skin

In addition to promoting better overall health, eating real food nourishes and helps protect your skin from the inside out. For instance, dark chocolate and avocados have been shown to protect skin against sun damage. Studies suggest that eating more vegetables, fish, beans and olive oil may help reduce wrinkling, loss of elasticity and other age-related skin changes. What's more, switching from a Western diet high in processed foods to one based on real food may help prevent or reduce acne.

8. Real Food Helps Lower Triglycerides

Blood triglyceride levels are strongly influenced by food intake. Because triglycerides tend to go up when you eat sugar and refined carbs, it's best to minimize these foods or cut them out of your diet altogether. In addition, including unprocessed foods such as fatty fish, lean meats, vegetables and nuts has been shown to significantly reduce triglyceride levels.

9. Real Food Provides Variety

Eating the same foods over and over can get old. It's

also healthier to include many different foods in your diet. There are hundreds of different real food options, including a wide variety of meat, fish, dairy, vegetables, fruits, nuts, legumes, whole grains and seeds. Make a point of regularly trying some real foods you've never eaten that look or sound interesting, such as kiwi, chia seeds, organ meats, kefir or quinoa. You might just find a few new favorites.

10. Real Food Costs Less in the Long Run

It's said that real food is more expensive than processed food, and in some ways this is true. A 2013 analysis of 27 studies from 10 countries found that eating healthier food costs about $1.56 more than processed food per 2,000 calories. However, in the long run, this difference is minimal compared with the cost of managing chronic lifestyle diseases such as diabetes and obesity. For instance, a 2012 study found that people with diabetes spend 2.3 times more on medical supplies and health care than people who don't have diabetes. So real food is more expensive in the short-term, but way cheaper in the long run --

because junk food costs you twice.

11. Real Food Is High in Healthy Fats

Unlike trans fats and processed fats found in vegetable oils and spreads, most naturally occurring fats are incredibly healthy. For example, extra virgin olive oil is a great source of oleic acid, a monounsaturated fat that promotes heart health.Coconut oil contains medium-chain triglycerides, which have been shown to increase fat burning and assist with weight loss. Long-chain omega-3 fatty acids help fight inflammation and protect heart health. Fatty fish, such as salmon, herring and sardines, are excellent sources of these fats .Other real foods that are high in healthy fats include avocados, nuts, seeds and whole-milk dairy.

12. Real Food May Reduce Disease Risk

Making real food part of your lifestyle may help reduce your risk for a number of chronic diseases.

Eating patterns based on whole, unprocessed foods — including the Mediterranean diet — have been shown to reduce the risk of heart disease, diabetes and metabolic syndrome.In addition, several large observational studies link a balanced diet with a high intake of fruits and vegetables to a decreased risk of cancer and heart disease.

13. Real Food Contains Antioxidants

Antioxidants are compounds that help fight free radicals, which are unstable molecules that can damage your body's cells. They are found in all real foods, especially plant foods like vegetables, fruits, nuts, whole grains and legumes.

Fresh, unprocessed animal foods also contain antioxidants, but their levels are generally much lower than in plants. For instance, egg yolks contain lutein and zeaxanthin, which help protect against eye diseases such as cataracts and macular degeneration.

14. Real Food Is Good for Your Gut

Eating real food may be beneficial for your gut microbiome, the bacteria that live in your digestive tract. Indeed, many real foods function as prebiotics — food that your gut bacteria ferment into short-chain fatty acids. In addition to promoting gut health, these fatty acids may improve blood sugar control and provide other health benefits. Real food prebiotics include garlic, asparagus and cocoa. For an extensive list of prebiotic foods, read this article.

15. Real Food May Help Prevent Overeating

A high intake of processed and fast foods has been linked to overeating, particularly in those who are overweight. By contrast, real food doesn't contain the sugars and flavorings found in processed foods that help drive overeating.

16. Real Food Promotes Dental Health

Healthy teeth may be another benefit of a real food

lifestyle that's low in sugars and refined carbs. Sugar and refined carbs promote dental decay by providing food for the plaque-causing bacteria that live in your mouth. The combination of sugar and acid in soda is especially likely to cause decay. Cheese seems to help prevent cavities by increasing pH and hardening tooth enamel. One study found that eating cheese dramatically improved enamel strength in people with limited saliva production due to radiation treatment for cancer. Green tea has also been shown to protect tooth enamel. One study found rinsing with green tea significantly reduced the amount of erosion that occurred when people drank soda and brushed their teeth vigorously.

17. Real Food May Help Reduce Sugar Cravings

A diet based on real food may also help reduce cravings for sweets, such as cake, cookies and candy. Once your body adjusts to eating whole, unprocessed foods, cravings for sugary foods could become infrequent and even disappear altogether. When you limit or avoid processed foods and high-sugar foods, eventually your taste buds adapt and learn to appreciate real food more.

18. Eating Real Food Sets a Good Example

In addition to improving your own health and well-being, eating real food can help the people you care about stay healthy as well. Leading by example can help encourage better eating habits for your family members. It's also a good way to help your kids learn about good nutrition.

19. Eating Real Food Gets the Focus off Dieting

A dieting mentality isn't good over the long term. It makes you focus on the number on the scale too much.Nutrition is about way more than just dieting. It is also about feeling good, having enough energy and being healthy. Focusing on real food instead of dieting can be a much healthier, more sustainable and enjoyable way to live. Instead of focusing too much on weight loss, let weight loss come as a natural side effect of a better diet and improved metabolic health.

20. Real Food Helps Support Local Farmers

Purchasing produce from farmers' markets, along with meat and dairy products from local farms, supports the people who grow food in your community. In addition, these are often much fresher and less processed than the foods you get at the supermarket.

21. Real Food Is Delicious

In addition to all of the other reasons to eat real food, it truly tastes delicious. The amazing flavor of fresh, unprocessed food is undeniable. Once your taste buds have adjusted to real food, processed junk food simply can't compare.

CHAPTER THREE

Wellness

Wellness is much more than merely physical health, exercise or nutrition. It is the full integration of states of physical, mental, and spiritual well-being. The model used by our campus includes social, emotional, spiritual, environmental, occupational, intellectual and physical wellness. Each of these seven dimensions act and interact in a way that contributes to our own quality of life.

• Social Wellness is the ability to relate to and connect with other people in our world. Our ability to establish and maintain positive relationships with family, friends and co-workers contributes to our Social Wellness.

• Emotional Wellness is the ability to understand ourselves and cope with the challenges life can bring. The ability to acknowledge and share feelings of anger, fear, sadness or stress; hope, love, joy and happiness in a productive manner contributes to our Emotional Wellness.

• Spiritual Wellness is the ability to establish peace and harmony in our lives. The ability to develop congruency between values and actions and to realize a common purpose that binds creation together contributes to our Spiritual Wellness.

• Environmental Wellness is the ability to recognize our own responsibility for the quality of the air, the water and the land that surrounds us. The ability to make a positive impact on the quality of our environment, be it our homes, our communities or our planet contributes to our Environmental Wellness.

• Occupational Wellness is the ability to get personal fulfillment from our jobs or our chosen career fields while still maintaining balance in our lives. Our desire to contribute in our careers to make a positive impact on the organizations we work in and to society as a whole leads to Occupational Wellness.

• Intellectual Wellness is the ability to open our minds to new ideas and experiences that can be applied to personal decisions, group interaction and community betterment. The desire to learn new concepts, improve skills and seek challenges in pursuit of lifelong learning contributes to our Intellectual Wellness.

Physical Wellbeing

When we talk of physical wellbeing, we aren't talking simply about the fitness of the body. Physical wellbeing is a big umbrella under which physical fitness is also a crucial point.

Let me state a few examples, just to explain this point better.

1. A 35 year old man. Living in one of the best cities in the world. Educated at the best school has a job, most people at his age can only dream of. He's married, with two kids and a beautiful home. Big cars, foreign vacations, fancy dinners, parties, etc. are part of his routine life.

This man is very healthy too. Doesn't eat unhealthy

food often, drinks but never exceeds his limit, doesn't smoke, doesn't do drugs, has absolutely no illness. Moreover, he exercises every day and also runs the city marathon.

In short, perfect life!

One day, he was crossing the street, going from his office to the restaurant across the road. He was meeting his lovely wife for lunch. He spotted her and waved with a smile. But that's when it happened.

He felt a searing pain running down his chest, through his left hand and he collapsed in the middle of the busy street. Two hours later, he was declared dead at the local hospital.

• Question - What happened? And why?

2. 50 year old housewife. Mother of two beautiful children and wife of a businessman. She spent her days doing what made her happy.

Every morning she'd leave for an orphanage and teach the children. Then she'd go to meet her friends or foundation members who helped run her

NGO.After a happy chit-chat and lunch, she'd go to her book club or wine tasting or one of the numerous activities she'd enrolled in. By evening she returned home to cook a lovely meal for her family. And the day ended with fun and laughter. Perfect!

Two weeks after her 25th wedding anniversary, she fainted in the orphanage and died of a haemorrhage.

• Question - Why? What went wrong? I have a whole lot of such stories that are shocking and mysterious. But the reason we need to analyze these cases carefully is for two reasons.

• Both these people, had seemingly happy and good lives. They were truly happy with their world and the people in it.

• Both these people, are not very different from how we are or wish to be one day.

Now, do you see why it is so serious?

In the examples given above, the man, had a perfect life. But he also had an ideal job. And no ideal job comes without stress. That was what caused his heart attack. As for the lady, she had a completely clean medical report, as far as physical health was concerned. But her psychiatrist revealed, that she had been severely depressed due to loneliness and that is why she kept herself so busy. Her constant running around, proved too much for her body to take.

We've made it a habit to let small instances in our life, pass by, assuming they aren't really important. We make a huge issue of a heart attack, a migraine or hyper-tension. But we seem to be okay with the unexplained tiredness, sore body, muscle spasms, unexplained headaches, etc. For us, these are day-to-day things.

And honestly, why shouldn't they be?. Who has time to live life worrying about every single papercut?.

BUT.

Would you worry if that papercut, wouldn't stop bleeding? Would it be enough to catch your attention? Or would it really take something like, collapsing or fainting, to finally make you realize that everything, is far from okay!

Physical wellbeing, is that scale or measure, which gives you a better idea of whether everything is really okay or not. It is the difference between being truly healthy and healthy by definition.

What is Physical Wellbeing?

• Physical wellbeing, is a combination of good physical, mental and emotional health. It is the result of the combination of all components, individually included in other forms of wellbeing.

• Simply being physically fit or emotionally strong or mentally well isn't enough.

• Physical wellbeing is the ultimate form of wellness achieved from all departments of human health put together. It is the larger picture of wellness.

Although it would be impossible to write everything about physical wellbeing, I think we should all make note of these specific markers so that we know when there is a red alert and what we can do to avoid them.

Signs of distress

• Excessive fatigue. Feeling more tired than usual and

more often

• Unexplainable headaches, sudden shooting pain, which later goes away.

• Dizziness when standing up and walking up or down stairs.

• Extreme anger or getting upset very easily.

• Inability to control emotions: Crying a lot.

• Excessive hunger or Loss of appetite.

• Sweating excessively.

These are just some of the many symptoms you may see. A very interesting symptom also includes, the need to work out a lot. It seems strange, but some people have a tendency to workout 2 or 3 times a day. That seems normal, but is sometimes not really normal. Remember, anything in excess is harmful.

Now let's take a look at what we can do to ensure wellbeing.

Measures to ensure Physical Wellbeing

• Drink plenty of water. Keep re-hydrating every half hour.

• Exercise regularly. Decide intensity based on your height and weight.

• Exercise in moderation. Don't overwork yourself.

• Have a meal that includes a good amount of proteins and carbs alike.

• Do NOT exclude fats from your diet entirely. That is harmful.

• Eat meals at regular intervals. Preferably 6 small meals a day.

• Take a break from work or studies. Never work at a stretch, 4 hours or more.

• Do things you enjoy doing, pursue hobbies and make them priorities

• Go out into the open and get a good amount of sunlight.

• Never stay locked up indoors all day long.

• Listen to calming music and watch light entertainment.

• Practise yoga or meditation or both! More the better.

• Make an effort to stay positive in general. Think happy, stay happy.

Mental Wellbeing

When it comes to mental wellbeing, there is a tendency to talk purely in terms of mental health. There is a preconceived notion that the lack of any mental illness, is defined as mental wellbeing. This is absolutely untrue. Just like not having any physical or physiological disease, doesn't make you fit; not having any mental diseases, doesn't make you mentally well.

Let's understand mental wellbeing in depth.

What is Mental Wellbeing?

• Mental wellbeing is a situation, where an individual is able to deal effectively with the stresses of life and contribute to society, without any pressures, emotional or otherwise.

• Mental wellbeing is more of an inclusive concept. Here the absence of mental illness, objectivity and productivity are all combined to measure the mental wellness of a person.

The World Health Organization in its comprehensive definition of health, stated, "Health is a state of complete physical, mental and social well-being and not merely the absence of disease or infirmity." This means, not having a disease doesn't make you healthy. What makes you healthy is a complete state of wellbeing. This is also what applies to the concept of mental wellbeing.

Not having any mental illness, does not mean there is mental wellbeing. Whenever we talk of mental wellbeing, we are in fact talking about the overall package. Unless a person has clarity of thought, objective decision making ability, productivity, etc. we cannot say that the person is mentally healthy.

A common error to be taken note of, is that mentally well and mentally sound are not the same thing! They are different in definition, not only medically, but also legally. A person who is mentally sound may not be mentally well. He may be highly disturbed.

Let us now take a look at some of the common mental illnesses or disorders and understand what they imply.

1. Depression

The most commonly known mental disorder, is also used as a term very synonymously with extreme sadness.

Depression is a state of low mood and aversion to activity that can affect a person's thoughts, behaviour, feelings and sense of well-being. People with a depressed mood can feel sad, anxious, empty, hopeless, helpless, worthless, guilty, irritable, ashamed or restless

(Note: Just to be clear, you are not depressed if you exhibit these symptoms alone.

Depression is something that only a qualified psychologist or psychiatrist can diagnose. The reason I am stressing this, is simple because we have a tendency to self-diagnose.)

2. Anxiety

It is a state of inner turmoil, where a person tends to feel an extreme sense of discomfort, guilt and becomes restless.

A person with an anxiety disorder, often makes up scenarios, without even realising that they are not real. Negative thoughts start to breed and a person loses calm easily.

3. Mood Disorders

Mood swings of extreme range are seen in this scenario. A person with mood disorders, is often unable to find a rational level between mania and depression (Mania - extremely high end Depression - extremely low end of emotion)

4. Obsessive Compulsive Disorder (OCD)

OCD is the inability to control the urge to perform a certain activity. It is more than often an activity which becomes a routine habit, which the person then finds impossible not to do.

OCDs can be as ordinary as the need to wash ones

hand every few minutes to dangerous ones like the need to self-harm.

5. Phobias

In simple terms FEAR. A phobia is an extreme fear which stops a person from performing certain activities or dealing with certain situations. So claustrophobia, makes people feel suffocated in a crowd, etc.

As per WHO, the well-being of an individual is encompassed in the realization of their abilities, coping with normal stresses of life, productive work and contribution to their community. Even if you think about it logically, it makes sense. We wouldn't look at a person who, has really high potential and is doing a really menial job or gets very upset about really trivial issues or does not get involved in some social activity, as a mentally well or happy person.

But, this also does not mean that a person who is always smiling and very affable and does social service, is actually happy! They say that people who smile the widest are the saddest. That is why it becomes essential to ensure mental wellbeing.

Let us now look at some of the best ways to ensure mental wellbeing.

1. Connect with people

With the advent of technology, if there is one thing we lost, it is the humane touch to our relationships. We have to remember that no matter how advanced the technology gets, the power that personal connections have, is unmatched. It is essential for mental wellbeing, that this connection with people takes place. When we talk to people we allow them to share our joys & sorrows. This impacts our mental wellbeing immensely.

2. Get a life-coach

From time to time, we all need a little bit of push. A little cheering to help us move on and get on with life. A life coach can help us leave behind our troubles and actually find the mental peace we so desire. It is always good to get some motivational advice and guidance. The mind clears up and we feel better.

3. Contribute to society

Doesn't have to be hours of social service. But a few hours a week or even if you can do something over the weekend, it can be very good for you. When you give back to society, it creates a sense of self-worth. We always feel better when we are in a position to give. It is human tendency. Contributing in any small way, can bring positive feelings.

4. Challenge yourself

Never mollycoddle yourself. Always give yourself challenging tasks and keep raising the bar. Your mind needs to feel challenged. Otherwise a sense of worthlessness and hopelessness kicks in.

So keep yourself active and up to any task at hand. Mental wellbeing comes only when there is satisfaction. What better satisfaction than completing challenges?!

5. Take it easy

Just because I said challenge yourself, don't put yourself into undue pressure. You have your own constraints. Never overestimate your strengths. This makes you set unrealistic goals. When these goals doesn't get fulfilled, the mind feels low and demotivated. Mental wellbeing is impossible without positivity. So always allow yourself some space. Take it easy on yourself.

6. Notice your surroundings

It may not always seem so, but this world is a pretty amazing place. Whenever you feel like there is a lack of balance, just look around yourself. Take notice of what is happening around you. The mind will become alert and it will come up with productive solutions to problems. Mental wellbeing, has as one of its components, productivity. Pay close attention to your surroundings.

Most importantly, live in the here and now. It is absolutely foolish, to miss a beautiful today, in hopes of a better tomorrow. Enjoy the moment.

7. Ask for help

There is no shame in not being able to stay 100% in control, all the time. There is no such thing as perfection. Nobody is perfect and neither are you. So if at some point you feel out of control, just go and ask for help. Doesn't have to be a doctor on the first go. You could talk to a friend, a favourite teacher, your parents, a counsellor or anyone! But ask for help when you need it.

Mental wellbeing is much easier to achieve when you have people you can go to for help.

Health and Wellness Tips with A Long Fitness Life

our health is your wealth. A healthy man is a wealthy man, literally. You may think of a tycoon who owns so much material wealth but their health troubles them. What is the point of all the material wealth if you cannot enjoy it? The money spent on doctors could have been channelled in other better avenues. Similarly, ever thought of how quick an employee gets replaced at work? You probably fell ill or a colleague passed on. The job vacancy goes up no sooner than the bad news leaves your mind.

Therefore, it is important that you take care of your health. It is with this in mind, we have noted down these health tips. There are simply recommendations. We are free to do more or less, as per what we desire.

1. Drink Water

This may sound cliché but it is very important. Top of the list in good health tips to practise is staying hydrated. The human body functions mainly on water. Take a person who is fasting, they can do away with food but they are allowed to take water. Water keeps you alert and keeps your body functional. At times, people have headaches simply because of dehydration. However, most people are quick to take paracetamol tablets. It is recommended that you take between 6 - 8 glasses of water every day. Stay hydrated and you definitely will remain rejuvenated.

2. Work out

Among daily health tips that we should not

compromise is working out. Now, you don't need to have a gym membership. Life is not as complicated. We all want to have the gym membership but what if you don't? You can simply buy a skipping rope and put in the cardio at home. Get a comfortable pair of trainers and have a morning or evening run. If that's too much, walk. If you own a pet, this can be ideal timing for you to bond.

3. Meditate

The career woman today has so much going on in her daily activities. She ought to be a wife at home, mother and deliver at work. It is very easy to lose yourself when so much is expected of you. Among the health tips for women would be embracing meditation. Most people say they don't have time for such but if it is important, you find time for it. Take time alone and just get lost in your positive thoughts. Visualize or even take part in yoga. You take control of your emotional health particularly which is very important.

4. Sleep well

Sleep is a very debatable subject. Some people prescribe 8 hours of sleep while others prescribe 6 hours. In the same line of thought, you hear of very successful people who sleep for 4 hours and are very functional. Therefore, my recommendation is sleep well. It is not the quantity but quality of sleep that counts. If you sleep for 10 hours and it's a noisy place, you won't rest well. You can however sleep for 2 hours in a very serene environment and get up very energetic. It is the quality that counts, not the quantity.

A power nap in the afternoon is said to keep one youthful. I don't know how true it is but there could be truth to it. What I know is that when you feel sluggish in the afternoon, a power nap goes a long way. There is no point of dragging through your tasks yet you can just sleep for ten minutes and be rejuvenated. However, do not be a serial afternoon sleeper and call it a power nap. That is outright laziness.

5. Eat well

Among the good health tips to practise on a daily is

your diet. Having a balanced diet is very important. Your body will not lack anything. Similarly, with food it is the quality and not quantity that matters. You may eat so much but your body will only take up what it needs. That roast beef can be very tempting but your body will only take up the amount of protein needed. Just have the appropriate serving for you. What is not used up ends up being fat in your body.

6. Laugh more

As absurd as it sounds, this is the easiest good health tip you can utilise. We live in a world where everybody is focused on getting things done. People no longer savour the taste of good food. People can't smell well brewed coffee. It is sad. People's moods are at an all time low. To avoid this, just afford a good laugh each day. Find humour in the little things. If laughing is tedious, smile. You never know who you will smile at and they will have a great day just because of your smile.

7. Socialise

Perhaps you are wondering what this means? In the

office setting, people don't necessarily socialise. Everyone is doing what brought them there and are quick to head home as soon as they are done. Not many people would say they are close to their colleagues. We don't know what challenges our colleagues may be facing at home. Similarly, people don't know if you have challenges.

CHAPTER FOUR

Natural Secrets To Healthy Looking Skin

As a person ages, a lot of changes occur in his anatomy. Most of these changes are unwanted as brought about by the seemingly common goal of the peoples of the world to preserve their youth. A perfect example of this is skin aging. Wrinkles, black marks, flakes and many other skin irregularities are avoided by many as it is considered as unhealthy and unattractive. This is the reason why secrets to healthy looking skin are sought by many.

Studies show that skin care is most effective if started from within. Cosmetics may only help one hide the irregularities, but the skin itself must be nourished from inside out. One of the many secrets to healthy looking skin is to know that genuine skin care must commence from regulating the food we eat everyday.

A proper diet will have a more lasting effect to your skin than cosmetics.

One good diet is 'fiber-loading'. A high fiber diet through eating lots of whole grains aids in eliminating toxins from your body which have adverse effects to your skin. Whole grains are also very good sources of anti-aging antioxidants. Therefore, instead of having your pasta and cookies, try having whole grains instead.

Another one of the many secrets to healthy looking skin is eating more fish. Fish has Omega 3 fatty acids which are found to lessen the risk of having skin cancer. Two servings of fish per week are just enough to provide your body with enough Omega 3 to ensure healthier skin. But of course, you can choose to have more.

Incorporating vegetable oil in your diet will also be a great help. Vegetable oil like sunflower oil and olive oil has a good amount of linoleic acid which prevents dry and flaky skin. It will moisturize your skin from within so you won't need to apply body lotion and body cream every now and then.

Eating citrus fruits is also one of the most advisable amongst the many secrets to healthy looking skin. As everyone knows, citrus fruits are rich in Vitamin C which is involved in collagen-formation. Collagen is a protein which acts as a bonding agent to tissues, thus keeping your skin firm and helps avoid wrinkles. So take more oranges, grapefruits, broccoli and bell peppers. They're good for you.

Looking Younger the Natural Way

I find that age is really first a matter of mind. Do not believe that you must show the signs of aging. Do not be with people who constantly complain about aches, pains, medications,etc. Make it your passion to be well and healthy. It all starts with you.

Simple things like drinking enough water are important. We need to be certain that we are well-hyrdated each day. Drinking coffee, juices, and soda pop is not true hydration; we need purified water and mineralized waters to help sustain true health. If you are eating foods that are denatured, over-processed, salted, smoked, and sweetened you might consider upgrading your food choices. By eating foods that are rich in vitamins, minerals, proteins and enzymes you will give your body more of what it needs to be vibrant. Visit a holisitc doctor who can help guide your personal wellness plan.

Eat foods from every color of the rainbow each week; colored sherbet and jellos don't count. Be sure to have red, orange, yellow, green, blue, and violet foods -both fruits and veggies. Cut back on alcohol and all sweets too. If you smoke please stop. Eating a wide variety of foods is important.

Get outside and allow your body to absorb some natural sunlight while you walk or bike or play some sport. Just walking at a fast pace is really wonderful exercise if you do it consistently through the week. So many of us are office-bound and drive much too often. What will sitting too long do for you? Nothing but bring illness! We must move in every way including moving our bowels to keep your body vibrant.

As far as keeping your skin as free from deep wrinkles as possible, including anti-oxidants in your daily diet. Look for richly colored natural foods and add an anti-oxidant supplement. Be sure that you take digestive enzymes as you age to help stimulate your metabolism and help your body rid itself of waste.

Apply a 100% natural oil after your shower. Be sure that you do not over consume refined carbohydrates, fried foods, and junk foods.

Another important component to looking and feeling more youthful than your actual age is to engage in activities that bring true inner peace. For some this may mean meditation, for others prayers or music or sitting still by a quiet lake or stream. Even sexual activity helps to bring inner peace when you are in love. The connection between two loving beings is a wonderful way to bring balance of body mind and spirit.

During your hectic day take a moment or two and

just mentally inhale that which you thoroughly adore; this could be a person, place, thing, an emotion such as the feeling of joy, the exhilaration of winning a contest, having millions of dollars suddenly fall into your lap, or anything else that brings you personal satisfaction. When you place yourself in the position to experience inner peace and joy you actually uplift your personal resonance, or the vibe that you send out to the world. When we send out beauty and joy and peace and honesty we will begin to sense those very same things returning to us.

Next, exhale all of the things you no longer need or want as part of you. Exhale fear, worry, grief, sadness, feelings of abandonment, shame, guilt, dishonesty, violations, anger, impatience, and all negative memories that have hurt you in some way. Let all of the people who have hurt you flow away from you and into this black box---they are not harmed just transformed into a more wonderful and loving person.

As you imagine letting go of all of the things that burden you each day try to be clear about what they are. In your mind's eye as you identify what has hurt you or someone else, let them gather and then see these things as black streams or gray streams or blobs that are moving away from you. See them flowing effortlessly into a large black box that is suspended in the air a distance from you. Once they hit the box they dissipate instantly and become sparkling white lights that gently return to you bringing wonderful feelings, filling you with exactly what you were needing at that moment.

When we are children we do not judge our actions or our emotions, we just act and we feel. Somewhere along the line we may be molded into thinking that something is good or bad, or that we may be good or bad so we stop doing certain things or we stop feeling to one degree or another. Boys are often told to hold in their emotions because they would be considered weak if shown. Girls are told not to be so emotional because it makes people feel uncomfortable. Try to reclaim those joyful moments by going to that place in your mind where you once experienced joy and allow your mind to recreate that feeling for you.

Mastering the practice of experiencing inner peace is something I hope everyone can accomplish; it is an exquisite space and one that brings such lovely balance of body, mind and spirit.

Other things that will help you slow down your personal aging: Being outside with nature, walking the beaches, hiking the mountains, looking at wildlife, taking warm baths in epsom salt, deep breathing exercises, doing one new thing a day, being with uplifting friends and family members, eating live foods that have life-giving energy more often, holding your favorite pet, being around children and watching them enjoy life, not cooking your food too long or at high temperatures, wearing clothes that allow your body to breathe. Take care of your body from your hair to the soles of your feet. Perhaps massage therapy will get your circulation going and that is paramount to good health.

Make whatever you choose to eat of the highest quality possible. It is said that when we are grateful for our food it will balance the molecular structure. A Japanese Doctor by the name of Masaru Emoto did a beautiful scientific study proving that water crystals align when we say a prayer or feel grateful and the chosen language didn't matter. Check that out on line. So being grateful for life, for all that you have, will also uplift you and others.

Choose your thoughts wisely. If you check your mind-chatter you may find that you are not your own best friend. If you are mentally sabotaging yourself please begin to change that mental movie. Try saying good things to yourself and about yourself. We must first learn how to love ourselves before we can truly love others. Write a list of all of your good traits. Say them aloud and write them into your mental script. Program yourself to be youthful.

Each day when I look in the mirror I say "You look 35!" I certainly am much older, however, the more you say things like this, the more the subconscious mind must act to create it. So get to work in the mirror starting today. Don't allow yourself to say horrible things about your body and don't let anyone else influence you about how you view yourself. It isn't always easy to let go of hurtful things other people may say, but it is important that you begin to take control of your health and it all starts with A THOUGHT!

Do things that make you laugh every day. Play a game with children. Watch how they have mastered the art of truly "playing" a game. They immerse themselves in game playing; so honest. Participate in in things that you love to do such as playing a musical instrument, dancing, boating, painting, singing, joining a non-for-profit group, visiting the museums, a ball park, or other activities that bring joy.

Every evening before bed practice inhaling youth and vibrance. Inhale joy and peace. Mentally see your body getting younger and try to feel it happening. Sense your skin tightening and becoming more elastic, feel your body fat shrinking, your eyes sparkling, your mind sharpening and your energy increasing.

CHAPTER FIVE

Choosing the Right Food for Health and Nutrition

Great health is only achievable by eating the right food for nutrition. It is apparent that everyone desires to feel great, energetic, and prevent common infections. However, without the right nutrition basics this is hardly achievable. Meal planning also enables someone to avoid junk food and encourages a consistent Intuitive nutritional therapy.

Health and nutrition tips

Planning a Intuitive nutritional therapy is the first step to nutritious eating. One cannot easily do this on the go; it takes discipline and small manageable steps. Start by thinking of the diet in terms of color rather than being overly concerned about the amount of calories intake. Fruits and vegetables are very colorful and useful in many recipes making the food more appetizing and palatable. These are the foundation of healthy eating and constitute highly required minerals vitamins and antioxidants

Nutrition improvement begins by making slow changes in one's eating habits and over time, getting accustomed to eating healthy. These can include measures liking switching from conventional butter to cooking with olive oil. Another very important ingredient in a diet is the use of water and exercise. Water flushes out waste from the system while exercise helps in improving metabolism and increased blood flow to the whole body.

It is important to eat a balanced diet that always includes proteins, carbohydrates, vitamins, minerals, fiber, and fat for sustainable health and nutrition. One does not have to think of some food as being off limits, however all food should be eaten in moderation and in the right quantities. What one needs to do if they have been eating unhealthy foods, for example salty and sugary foods, is to start reducing the intake slowly. The body gradually adjusts to the new alternative and soon eating healthy becomes a habit.

Starting the day with breakfast, followed by small frequent meals for the rest of the day, is energizing and increases metabolism. Whenever one has the opportunity, they should buy fresh produce from local farmers.

Healthy carbohydrates and whole grains for good nutrition

Carbohydrates and fiber rich foods for nutrition are very important as they give us energy to go through the day. These are available in whole grains and are rich in antioxidants and phyotochemicals, which are helpful in protecting against coronary heart diseases, diabetes and some forms of cancer. They digest more slowly keeping one feeling fuller for longer while keeping insulin and blood sugar levels at a healthy low. However, one needs to differentiate between the good and unhealthy carbohydrates. The good carbohydrates constitute of whole grains, legumes, fruits, and vegetables, while unhealthy carbohydrates constitute refined sugars and flour.

Tips to help you feed your hunger and not your emotions

Imagine if eating were as simple as, say, refueling a car. You'd fill up only when an indicator nudged towards E, you couldn't possibly overdo it or else your tank would overflow, and you'd never, ever dream of using it as a treat.

Instead, for many of us, eating is anything but straightforward. What starts out as a biological necessity quickly gets entangled with different emotions, ideas, memories and rituals. Food takes on all kinds of meanings — as solace, punishment, appeasement, celebration, obligation – and depending on the day and our mood, we may end up overeating, undereating or eating unwisely.

It's time for us to rethink our relationship with food :

1. Reconnect with your hunger.

So many things drive us to eat — it's noon and that means lunchtime, it's midnight and that means snack time, we're happy, we're anxious, we'd rather not bring home leftovers, we're too polite to say no, we're bored, and oh, wow, has someone brought in donuts?!?

Similarly, we suppress our appetite for a myriad of reasons — we're too busy, we're sad, we're mad, nobody else is eating, it's too early, it's too late, we're too excited.

Now try doing this: Eat only when you're hungry; stop when you're full.

Eve Lahijani, a Los Angeles-based dietician and a nutrition health educator at UCLA suggests that we think about our hunger and our fullness on a 0-10 scale, with 0-1 being famished and 9-10 being painfully stuffed (as in holiday-dinner stuffed). She says, "You want to begin eating when you first get hungry, and that correlates with the three or a four on the scale and [to stop] ... when you first get comfortably full, a six or seven on the scale."

The reason you shouldn't wait until you're starving (or, 0-2 on the scale) is because that's when people tend to make nutritionally unsound choices. If you've ever gone to the supermarket when you were ravenous, you probably didn't fill up your cart with produce; you gravitated towards the high-calorie, super-filling items.

Lahijani says, "It's also wise to eat when you first get hungry because you're more likely to enjoy your food [and] you're more likely to eat mindfully ... When you let yourself get too hungry, chances are, you're eating really fast and not really paying attention. In fact, one of the biggest predictors of overeating is letting yourself get too hungry in the first place."

2. Feed your body what it is craving.

When Lahijani was a stressed-out college and graduate student, her eating took one of two forms: she was either dieting or bingeing. As she says: "Whenever I was on a diet, the diet told me what to eat,"; while on a binge, she'd eat whatever was convenient or go all out on foods forbidden by her then-diet. Developing a different relationship with food meant stepping out of those patterns. "Instead of listening to others' opinions of what I should eat, I became silent and I tuned into my own body," she says. "I fed my body what it was craving."

It turns out Lahijani didn't crave junk food. She says, "I was actually tasting things for the first time, because my mind wasn't filled with judgment and guilt. I actually found that my body actually craved nurturing, nourishing foods like vegetables and fruits. I actually liked my sister's kale and quinoa salad."

3. Try not to use food as a reward or a punishment.

It's not surprising that we do this. After all, as children, we quickly learn that rejoicing and parties come with cake, while transgressions result in … no cake. But one of the great things about being an adult is, we can establish our own associations. By all means, let's continue to mark our birthdays with cake

— or with fresh fruit and a stockpot of homemade veggie chili if that's what you prefer. Or, celebrate in ways that have nothing to do with eating. You can set your own rules now.

When Lahijani's fraught feelings about food eased, she was surprised to find these effects go beyond eating. "What's really interesting is to see how making peace with food affected other areas of my life. As I learned how to listen to myself, I became better at listening to others, I became more empathetic," she says. "As I made a point to trust myself, I became more trusting in my relationships and more vulnerable, and as I became more loving to myself … I learned what it meant to love someone else."

CHAPTER SIX

Essential Component of Any Intuitive nutritional therapy

It is so important that we all eat Intuitive nutritional therapys, not only to feel good, but to look great as well. When we are not eating healthy, we do not look healthy. Our hair and skin look dull, our fingernails are brittle and our eyes look tired and lifeless. But when we are getting all of the nutrients we need in our diet, it really does show and you will not only look better, but you will feel a whole lot better too. There are three macronutrients that we all need in our diets in order to be healthy and actually, to survive. These macronutrients are carbohydrates, fats, and proteins and even with all of the bad things we hear about fat and carbohydrates, there are good ones and they are both necessary components of a Intuitive nutritional therapy.

What Is Protein?

Protein is an essential macronutrient and one that need to be a part of every Intuitive nutritional therapy. Protein is necessary for the growth and maintenance of our muscles and provides much of the energy that we need to get through our daily activities. Protein is made from chains of amino acids, of which there are two types: essential and non-essential. Essential amino acids are necessary to have in our systems and our bodies are not able to produce them. So, we must get the essential amino acids from dietary sources and there are all kinds that are great for any diet, including low calorie diets that are meant for weight loss.

There are eight essential amino acids: leucine, isoleucine, lysine, threonine, tryptophan, valine, methionine, and phenylalanine. Non-essential amino acids are those that the body is able to produce, therefore it is not necessary to get them from dietary sources. There are 14 non-essential amino acids in proteins: alanine, arginine, asparagine, aspartic acid, cysteine, cystine, proline, serine, taurine, glutamine, tyrosine, ornathine, glutamic acid, and glycene.

There are two types of protein, complete and incomplete. Complete proteins are proteins that contain all 22 of the essential and non-essential amino acids and can be found in all animal-based proteins, as well as soy. Incomplete proteins, which is what you will find with all plant-based proteins (except soy) do not contain all of the amino acids and in order to make sure that you get them all, you must eat a variety of the foods that contain some or most of the essential and non-essential amino acids.

Getting Enough Protein in Your Diet

If you have decided to add protein and other nutrients to your diet, it is important that you get your nutrients from the right dietary sources. There are all kinds of things you can eat that may have some nutrients, but they are not always good for you. This is why you really need to do your research and learn which foods are best for the type of diet you wish to follow, no matter if you want to lose weight, gain muscle, or just want to feel healthy and look great.

There are many good dietary sources of protein that are great for any diet, and if you eat the right protein rich snacks between meals, you will feel fuller and not feel the urge to snack on unhealthy treats. Of course, it is alright to have a treat now and again, as long as you are making sure that all of your nutritional needs are being met each and every day. There are two dietary sources of protein, animal and plant. All animal-based proteins are complete proteins and there are many that are not only diet friendly, but are extremely delicious too. A Intuitive nutritional therapy can include lean red meats, white meat poultry (breast meat), fish, low-fat dairy products, and eggs.

You can also get plenty of protein from plant-based proteins, although because they are incomplete, they need to be eaten in combination to get all of the proper nutrients. Some really healthy plant-based proteins you can add to your diet, even a weight loss diet, include whole grain breads and pastas, brown rice, nuts and seeds (unsalted), potatoes, broccoli, avocados, and much more.

What to Do When Your Diet Is Just Not Enough

There are going to be times in your life when you just can't get all of the nutrients you need from your diet. Sometimes, you are just far too busy to cook a meal, let alone sit down and eat it. Then of course there are times when you decide to stop and get take-out food and you definitely are not getting the nutrients you need with this kind of food. If you have kids who are fussy eaters, they may not be getting all of the nutrients that are vital to their growth and good health. So, with all of these things standing in your way, how can you be sure that you are always getting enough protein, as well as other nutrients and vitamins, in your diet every day? Supplements. There are all kinds of protein supplements available that will provide what you are missing in your diet. The key thing to remember is that they are not to be used all the time and you do have to make sure that you are eating some healthy food as well.

When you do decide to use protein supplements in your diet, you have a number of options to choose from. There are many different types of protein supplements, made from many different types of protein sources. Whey is a really popular protein supplement, for a number of reasons. It works quickly and is easy to digest, and it is one of the most inexpensive forms of protein supplements. Rice is another popular source of protein for supplements, because it is so easy to digest. Rice protein is hypoallergenic, so it is ideal for those who have food allergies or intolerances. Soy is another popular form of protein and is the only plant-based protein that is complete. One drawback to soy is that some people find it difficult to digest.

Vitamin B12: A Critical Component of a Healthy Diet

Vitamin B12 is also known as cobalamin. It is responsible for maintaining brain and nervous system health and aids in the production of blood. It is also needed for metabolism and DNA health. It is naturally found in liver, meat, milk products, eggs, cereal, barley, some algae, and bacteria. Since it contains cobalt, it is a red color. Half of the body's B12 is stored in the liver, which can store years worth of B12. It is recommended for adults to take 2 to 3 μg per day.

Pernicious anemia destroy stomach cells which produce intrinsic factor, which is needed to absorb vitamin B12. This type of anemia may cause a deficiency in vitamin B12. Some forms of B12 are used to treat cyanide poisoning. It is also used to treat optic neuropathy. Since vitamin B9 and B12 share many of the same responsibilities, it is harder to detect a B12 deficiency, especially since B9 is added to flour in most countries to prevent birth defects. It is also hard to detect a B12 deficiency since these symptoms match many other causes such as aging and atherosclerosis. With a B12 deficiency, more homocysteine is kept in the body, which causes damage to arteries. This leads to heart disease, heart attacks, and strokes since clotting occurs to repair the arteries. A lack of B12 also results in the irreversible deterioration of the spinal cord and nervous system, which is why a slight deficiency can show the symptoms of memory loss, depression with suicidal tendencies, mania, psychosis, paraphrenia complex which can develop into a wide range of mental diseases ranging from paranoia to schizophrenia, myelosis funicularis, and fatigue. If the deficiency affects the brain in any way, most of the time the damage is irreversible. Since it is needed to produce neurotransmitters in the brain, a deficiency can lead to depression.

Also, some antacids reduce the body's ability to absorb B12, leading to a deficiency. Those who have stomach, pancreas, and small intestine absorption issues may also be deficient in B12. Most of it is reabsorbed when it is used in digestion. Liver does a very good job of treating anemia, however iron seems to be a better way to treat anemia. Vitamin B12 has also been known to prevent Alzheimer's disease and psoriasis, a skin rash. Alcohol and nicotine will affect the absorption of many vitamins including B12 and should not be used everyday. Many medicines have a risk of increasing B12 deficiency including antibiotics, cholesterol medication, anticonvulsants, and antacids for the stomach and other parts of the body. Also, potassium affects the absorption of B12, which can lead to a deficiency.

CHAPTER SEVEN

The Process of Detoxification

You've made the decision to live a better, healthier lifestyle: you've eliminated the foods with the intention of saying no to disease and poor health; you're consuming more fresh fruits, vegetables, nuts, seeds, and grains in their natural state; you're on a dieting curriculum; and you're furthermore drinking lots of water and getting lot of sleep all night...

So why do you feel exhausted, rundown, and even sick every time?

It is called detoxification, and as a lifestyle exchange for the better is undertaken, some individuals will experience this in diverse degrees. But why does it take place? To take up this issue, we need to understand why we develop ailments every now and then, and what the body does to correct them. All ailments can be induced by these two foremost causes: toxicity and deficiency. Both are as result of our day to day feeding habits. Toxicity refers to a level of poison in the body from foods which have caused an acidic disequilibrium. These poisons are the by-products of consuming foods from animal sources, as well as sugar, salt, white flour products, caffeine, and other items which were modified from their first whole-food design (refined foods).

Deficiency is the state in which our body lacks Passable nutrients essential for the body's normal function, caused by the excessive consumption of foods which were refined or predominantly cooked until they are Rendered nutritionally incomplete.

When toxic foods are cut down, and we start the of intake of natural foods, especially fresh vegetable juices, the body is able to rebuild as well as cleanse itself. This domestic refining results in toxins/poisons being emptied into the bloodstream, this is what many individuals refer to as detoxification. During this process, you could experience a range of both physical and mental discomfort which will subside over a period, depending on the amount, degree, time spent consuming detoxifying diet. Eventually, as the "bad" gets eliminated and the "good" is deposit back in, symptoms start to abate, and the body starts functioning normally and return to good shape. Many individuals are encouraged to detoxify, or clean, the body initially, and later to rebuild the body. But wouldn't it be better to cleanse and nourish the body with valuable stuff from the very start with the intention of giving the body strength to rebuild and take up again to its normal function while it is furthermore refining? Therefore, it is essential to deal with both the toxicity and deficiency issues at the same time.

Why does detoxification occur?

The foremost function of the body is to create homeostasis - the state by which each part of the body is by the book balanced and in a state of normal function. Over the years, as our body homeostasis is upset due to lifestyle choices, the body starts to function in a constant mode of renovation and refurbishment. Working to keep you alive by all means possible. To accomplish this, the body tries to divest itself of the toxic elements with the intention of ridding itself of the toxins that has been built up in the system. If the body is unable to fully clean itself of the toxins, they could be stored deep surrounded by the tissues and cells. Unfortunately, it is as toxins are stored within the body that real destruction begins to occur in persons disease start to manifest. But as we commence making healthier nourishment and lifestyle choices, the body starts a refining process - eliminating the bad (toxins) and putting in the needed (natural nutrients) -and the areas damaged by stored toxins commence the rebuilding process.

The refining process has several avenues of purification:

1. Elimination through the bowels. One of the generally valuable issues to take up in detoxification is elimination. There are some indications that approximately 75-90% of people suffer from sluggish bowels. This can be a notification sign of greater health problems to occur. If toxins from our body (dead cells, dissipate products, and that.) are not eliminated quickly, they can be re-absorbed into the

body and hence lead to the upshot in the toxic buildup, which can ultimately result into the breakdown of the body and illness. Therefore, it is essential that bowel function be optimized in order to insure rapid and efficient dispersal of toxins.

2. Elimination through the skin. One way to help eliminate toxins is scrubbing off dry skin. For this process, the exhausted cells on the skin are brushed away. We lose close to two pounds of toxins all the time through our skin. Our skin is our leading organ and as such, as the bowels are not eliminating as they must, the toxins will try to leave the body anyway they could and the skin is one of such chance. This is why approximately anybody will develop rashes or spots as their body goes through a refining process.

3. Elimination through the lymph system. The lymph system is part of the immune system, and it assists the body in ridding itself of toxic elements; however, the lymph system does not flow through the body except the body acts. Thus, physical exercise is an essential element when it comes to dealing with symptoms of detoxification and rebuilding the immune system. An

exceptional way to move the lymph is through walking or rebounding for at least sixteen minutes daily.

4. Elimination through the mucous membranes. The mucous membranes enclose toxins and help to eliminate them from our system; however, if the mucous does not maintain a watery uniformity, the trapped toxins could become infectious now and again infection will develop. Consuming a passable amount of water (6-8 glasses every day) will help keep the mucous watery sufficient to enhance speedy passage of mucous.

What do you do when experiencing detoxification?

there are various symptoms of detoxification that could be manifested. Some indicators could be severe, such as flu-like symptoms, diarrhea, vomiting, and depression, but generally will be mildly irritating, and could include: headaches, fatigue, constipation, fever, skin rash, spots, bad temper, and lethargy, amongst others. The majority of individuals who change their feeding habits (natural food consumption) don't even realize that they undergoing the detoxification process. Others will notice mild refining or detoxification symptoms, such as fatigue, within a few days of making the change, while a very small percentage will experience significant detoxification signs weeks later. Each person is unique, and all individuals react in a unique way. As a matter of importance, we need to recognize detoxification as a clear process. It is one way the body can tell us it is working properly. Once we realize this we better understand and acknowledge why detoxification is occurring. There are various processes you could perform as an individual undergoes detoxification.

1: Do nothing and allow the body's detoxification process to run its way. The body will detoxify to the best of its ability. Generally, these detoxification episodes continue for about 3 - 7 days.

2: Slow down the refining process. Eat more cooked foods and cut back on the detoxifier this will normally results in an easing of the detoxification symptoms because the body is concentrating more of its energy on digesting and dealing with cooked foods than it is with refining and rebuilding.

3: Speed it up! Help the body to clean more quickly. This detoxification method entails eliminating solid foods; increasing water, intake fasting; and maybe even engaging in enemas or colonics! The symptoms won't disappear; instead, they could even intensify for a period. But as they are ended, they ordinarily wouldn't reoccur in the same fashion.

Foods That Help You Detox and Cleanse

More and more people are becoming aware of the mass assault on our food supply due to chemicals, pesticides and genetically modified foods all in the name of profit. While stock holders are happy, what about the millions of people who are nutritionally deficient and suffering with ailments and disease needlessly! The key to good health relies on the correct ratio of acid/alkaline balance in the body. How one achieves this is by eating 75% alkaline forming foods and 25% acid forming foods, preferably organic.

Acid Forming Foods

- All processed foods! This includes pastas, cakes, cookies, salad dressings etc.
- Meats, including Beef, pork, bird, fish, shellfish, eggs
- All dairy products, including butter, milk, cream, ice cream, cheese
- Nuts
- Sodas
- Caffeine, coffee, tea
- All breads
- Alcohol
- All foods with sugar
- Vegetables such as asparagus, sauerkraut, chickpeas, brussels sprouts
- Vinegar
- Lentils
- Plums, prunes, cranberries
- Alkaline Forming Foods

- Salad greens

- Fresh fruit

- Dried fruit such as raisins, dates, figs, apricots

- All sprouts

- All vegetables (except the ones listed above) Especially good are onions and garlic

- Citrus fruits (even though they are acidic, they have an alkalizing affect on the body)

- Good fats such as olive and flaxseed oil

- Honey, maple syrup and molasses

- Herbal teas

- Fresh fruit and vegetable juices

- Yogurt and sour cream

- Almonds, brazil nuts

If you look closely at the lists above you can get a pretty good idea of what you currently may be eating more of, whether acid or alkaline type foods. To get a more accurate measure you can buy ph strips from any drug store and see exactly where you are at and what you need to do create the optimum ph balance in your body.

In optimum health the body will naturally filter, cleanse, detox and extract nutrients efficiently.

If you find you are over acidic or alkaline you can take steps to repair the situation by switching over to the foods you should be eating on a regular basis.

Water is also extremely important in not only the cleanse cycle, but in normal daily function. You would be surprised at how many people are generally dehydrated and suffering needlessly with pain and fatigue, and it is a very easy fix. Drink up! Lots of water! You'll feel much better. (This is a major undiagnosed problem for seniors)

Benefits of a Detoxification Diet

here are some things you should know before starting such program. You may not need a detoxification diet if you are elderly or under weight. For pregnant or breast-feeding women or persons who are taking certain medication it would be advisable to check with their GP first, or better still visit a knowledgeable natural health practitioner. A detoxification diet is healthy when used as a short-term cleansing program. After that to continue and to get the best benefit would be to renew a long-term commitment into a healthy ongoing maintainable diet.

The Need for Detoxification

Some of the reasons why this type of diet has become more important is because of the changes and availability of unhealthy food over recent time, and the increase of toxins we are exposed to every day. This has become noticeable clear over the last decade or so in the increase of obesity and its health problems for people who are not aware of the dangers in some of today's foods. Therefore, detoxification diets have become more important and are more beneficial than in the past. There are many detox programs available today where we can target certain health issues. Probably one often used aspect of a detox is for those who struggle to lose weight. This is when the need for such a diet becomes a benefit because it emphasizes healthy food. Every day our body's cells are under attack from free radicals and toxins from processed high fat foods, pollution in every day household chemicals and even stress. All of this causes D N A cells breaking down and their ability to make healthier cells. Starved cells will not survive, just like your body needs food to survive the cells need nutrition to live. If your cells are not getting life-giving nutrients than they will slowly shrink and die off, becoming unhealthy and fast aging will increase. At that time many problems can arise. It can cause chronic pain, fatigue, excess water retention, it can affect memory and eyes. There are many reasons for the need of a detox diet, which can address a variety of health issues.

Detox for Weight Loss

For the purpose of weight loss this is probably one of the most important aspects of a detox especially for those who struggle to lose those extra few kilos or pounds. One of the main reasons is that this diet will help you to remove those bad influences in your diet because it emphasizes healthy food. More ever, the detox program focuses on removing stress and giving you the peace of mind you need. Stress is a crucial factor if you want to lose weight, and this is where a detox diet is the easiest way to lose weight naturally.

Improves Mental Focus

There are many who tried this diet reported an enhanced ability to concentrate better and as well increase in their creativity. According to recent studies performed, there is a strong head-body connection, so when your body feels good, your mind starts to react, and vice versa. As many things are improving in your body, this is the case when you start to feel better and lighter, at the same time your mind becomes healthier, clearer, and more active than ever before.

More Energy Less Headaches

If you are lacking of energy such detoxification program could bring back the energy and stamina. As food creates energy, what you eat in this diet will give you the energy you need, because some foods convert into energy better than other foods, such as processed meats, sweets or snacks. In general this diet will help increase the endorphin level in your body, giving you more energy and allowing you to focus on those daily more important tasks with ease. Many times headaches are becoming less or stop all together or you can experience less severe headaches by following this diet. A detoxification diet as such will be extremely helpful and of great benefit, especially if you have an unIntuitive nutritional therapyary lifestyle and are lacking of energy to finish all your tasks. In addition to the benefits outlined, this diet cleans out your colon, pancreas, kidney and liver. All this is helping your organs functioning properly and increases your overall health.

CHAPTER EIGHT

The Building Blocks of Your health

The saying, "You are what you eat" is more than a mere catch phrase or cliché. The reality is that what we become physically is significantly influenced by what we put into our bodies. Proper nutrition is getting what you need, the right amount of macronutrients, such as protein, carbohydrates and safe fats, plus micronutrients, including vitamins, minerals and essential fatty acids. By supplying our body each day with the elements of which it's composed, we can attain optimum health - provided that due attention is also given to our mind and spirit.

Every part of our body is fed and develops from the food we eat, food being nature's original remedy to activate our natural healing energies. Food fads may come and go, but the importance of a well-rounded diet and nurturing your body through healthful food never goes out of style. We can see this for ourselves; those who are more youthful and have abundant energy in most cases follow more wholesome diets, exercise regularly and follow a healthier lifestyle. People who are health-minded look it! They take responsibility for their lives and their choices, and it usually pays off with bright, clear eyes, glowing skin and full, healthy hair.

Conversely, those people who consume junk (processed/lifeless) foods and live unhealthy, sedentary lives are the ones who usually suffer from various health problems and are prone to premature aging. Of course there are people who are dealt a genetic royal flush. They can break all the rules in the book and nothing seems to affect the condition of their health, their energy or their appearance. Since life isn't fair, most of us are not part of that blessed minority.

We're all human, and what we don't understand we tend to criticize or ridicule. Most of us are like that, aren't we? I know I was leery and maybe even judgmental when I first heard about eliminating meat from my diet, cutting out junk food and eating plenty of fresh organic fruits and vegetables. However, implementing these changes made a dramatic and very positive difference

.The core building blocks of food are sugars, starch and oil. These three things provide our basic carbon and energy requirements. Different plants have unique levels and available proportions of these essential building blocks.

Seeds containing starch can have a descent amount of oil compared to oil seeds, which have no starch. Starch in the diet is usually provided by grains and vegetables, like potatoes.

Sugars freely available in sweet food are fructose, glucose, and sucrose. There is much to be read and learnt about these sugars beyond the scope of this article.

Oils in the diet are naturally obtained from foods with high oil content. Avocados are known for their high oil content. Nuts are another source of oils in the diet. We don't need to consume oil (cooking or otherwise) to receive adequate oils.

Vegetarians will passionately tell you we don't need meat in our diets to receive adequate Nutrition levels. The human body can happily and fundamentally gain its nutritional requirements from non-meat sources. Vegetarians know this and do it successfully. Many animal species eat nothing more than plant based nutrition.

There is ongoing debate about the nutritional levels of Organically grown food compared to food grown using modern traditional methods. One segment missing from these debates is the amount of pesticide residues on non-organic produce. The emphasis is focused only on the nutritional value.

Although scientific research and logical opinion differ, my logical view is that a plant will absorb the nutrients it requires regardless of their source. The important point ism, was the source real and natural or synthetic?

Organic, Natural food is grown with the idea that a

plant obtains its nutrition from nature. Plants have been growing successfully for centuries, long before man and science discovered a way to synthetically manufacture a fake version of nature.

The best way to determine if a plant or its fruit is nutritionally adequate is to observe the plant or fruit itself. If it looks healthy and delicious it most likely is. Plants show signs of inadequate nutrition by changes in their growth habit changes in leaf colour, poor fruit production or smaller than expected plant growth.

For maximum health benefits, look for food grown without the use of synthetic Pesticides. The look, feel and taste of the food will provide logical fact regarding the Nutritional value of it.

Healthy food will be naturally high in essential sugars, starch and oils needed for a healthy human diet.

Organically grown food often looks distorted or may have odd shapes. This does not have anything to do with the health of the plant or the food, it simply means the fruit was not grown for uniformity but rather quality and taste.

Tips on How to Take Control of Your Weight

1. Cleansing the body

This should be the first step for anyone embarking on a weight loss journey. This is a process of removing toxins from the body. The following are different ways of cleansing the body. These are:

a) Detox diets

b) Fasts

c) Colonic irrigation

a) Detox diets

Detoxification has been practiced for a long time by various cultures around the world. It involves resting cleaning and nourishing the body from the inside to the outside. This way, toxins are removed and eliminated and after that the body is fed with healthy nutrients. Detox helps you to renew your ability to maintain good health.

Despite their benefits, detox diets should be done carefully after consulting a doctor.

A good detox diet is one that nourishes your body with the right nutrients to keep our systems working smoothly and to aid in removing toxins from our bodies. Detox diets help the body's natural healing process by,

i) Resting the organs

ii) Stimulating body organs to remove toxins from the body

iii) Improving blood circulation

iv) Refueling the body with healthy nutrients

There are many detox diets in the market that involve extremely low calorie intake, which can rob the body of essential nutrients causing dehydration fatigue dizziness nausea and even colon damage. They also place the body in starvation mode, which, basically slows down your metabolic rate. These detox plans should be completely avoided.

b) Fasting

Fasting is a powerful therapeutic process that can help cleanse the body. Fasting basically means abstaining from food or drink. For body cleansing purposes, there are two different fasts, which also help with rapid weight loss.

i) Water fast

ii) Juice fasts

i. Water fast

This is the most grueling type of cleansing diet. During this fast, you can only take water. According to alternative health experts water fasts allow the body to heal and release all the toxins.

Water fasts should however not be done for long periods of time and they should be done only under the supervision of a doctor.

ii. Juice fast

Just like in water fast, a juice fast involves abstaining from food and drinking certain types of juices.

2. Reduce salt intake

Salt does not cause the human body to lose or gain fat. Consuming large quantities of salt can result into temporary weight gain. This is because salt contains sodium, which makes our bodies retain water. When there is excess sodium in our bloodstream water is needed to dilute its presence. This causes the body to retain 1.5 liters of water, which is equal to around 2-3 pounds. Switching to a low sodium diet can lead to the loss of the retained water and hence fast weight loss. However switching back to a high sodium diet could cause the weight to pile back on.

Reducing salt intake should be a long-term plan because it has more benefits to your health such as: reducing high blood pressure, lowering the chances of cancer and alleviating pre-menstrual symptoms among others.

Most people consume more salt than they actually need. It is recommended that an adult should consume 2.3 grams of sodium per day. This is around 6 grams of table salt in all the food consumed in entire day.

Tips on reducing salt intake

i) Buy fresh vegetables. When buying canned or

frozen vegetables, choose those that are 'plain' with 'no salt added'.

ii) Use fresh lean meat, poultry and fish. This is because a lot of sodium is used for processing meats.

iii) When cooking rice, pasta and hot cereals, avoid adding salt to them.

iv) Rinse canned food such as tuna to reduce the amount of sodium

v) Use homemade or low sodium broth when cooking

vi) Add herbs, spices, fruit juices and vinegars to flavor food rather than using salt.

vii) Snack on fresh fruits rather than snacks with high amounts of sodium such as salt crackers and chips.

viii) Condiments with a lot of salt such as ketchup and mustard should be used sparingly.

ix) When eating out, request your food to be prepared with a little salt.

x) Be careful when using salt substitutes as some may

contain large quantities of salt.

3. Increase water intake

Drinking water is one of the easiest activities that you can include in your weight loss plan. Unlike abstaining from tempting high calorie foods and going to the gym, drinking water requires very little will power.

Water and weight loss are a great pair. This is because our bodies are made up 60% to 70% water. Our bodies need water to function well and these functions are essential for weight loss.

This is how water helps in weight loss:

i) Kidneys require water to function properly. When there is insufficient water in the body for the kidneys to use, the liver has to step in and help. This causes a problem because one of the functions of a liver includes breaking down excess fat. When this happens, the liver becomes less efficient in breaking down fat.

ii) Water assists in the digestion and absorption of

food. Not consuming enough water means that the food you eat does not benefit you fully. It could also lead to constipation.

iii) Drinking ice-cold water could lead to burning more calories.

iv) Blood consists of around 83% water. Blood transports oxygen and nutrients throughout our bodies. When we are dehydrated our blood becomes thicker making it function less efficiently. This makes you feel fatigued and tired and therefore less active.

v) When we drink water we fill up the stomach. This helps in reducing cravings and appetite. Drinking water before meals will help you to consume fewer calories.

4.As the saying goes, breakfast is the most important meal of the day. This is especially true when you are trying to lose weight. Eating breakfast can aid in weight loss in the following ways.

i) Increasing metabolism

Good metabolism plays an essential role in weight

loss. After about 12 hours of not eating, your body goes into a state of a mild fast, as if no food is available. When you avoid eating until lunchtime, that could mean staying hungry for up to 18 hours. This leads to your body trying to conserve energy and therefore slowing down metabolism instead of working at its peak and burning more calories. When you eat a healthy breakfast your metabolic rate increases causing the body to work harder and burn plenty of calories.

ii) Keeps you motivated

A nutritious breakfast provides you with enough energy to keep you motivated and active the whole day. Eating a healthy breakfast will enable you to stay active throughout the day, increase your energy levels and hence give you a higher chance of burning calories.

You are more likely to exercise when you do not feel exhausted and sluggish the whole day.

iii) Helps in making healthy choices

After eating a healthy breakfast chances are you will

make healthy choices throughout the day. When you skip breakfast, you will start feeling hungry later and opt for a sugar loaded quick fix.

How to eat breakfast for weight loss

i) Eat breakfast as soon as you wake up. This will not only jump-start your metabolism but it will make sure that you do not feel starved later on in the day.

ii) Do not eat food that will lead to a midmorning crash. Instead, eat food that is high in fiber and protein. These foods digests slowly making sure you stay satisfied and energized the whole day.

iii) Make sure you do not over indulge as this could leave you feeling tired and bloated.

5. Eat small portions frequently

A dieter's biggest enemy is hunger. A sudden drop in blood sugar level causes hunger pangs. Eating small frequent meals is very beneficial to your weight loss goals. Dividing your daily calorie requirements into small 5-6 meals a day ensures that hunger pangs are kept at bay. Reasons of eating small portions frequently are as follows:

i) Suppressing appetite

Eating smaller meals more often plays a major role in suppressing appetite and cravings. Eating healthy whole foods frequently, and in small portions ensures that you stay satisfied and therefore you will be less likely to binge on high calorie carbs.

ii) Keeping up energy

Small and frevent meals will also help in keeping your energy high. 5-6 small meals at regular intervals help to keep the blood sugar steady. This way you will be feeling energized making you more active and burning a lot of calories. It will also help prevent sugar cravings.

iii) Stimulating your metabolism

When you deny your body food for a long time, it automatically switches to starvation mode. During starvation mode the body slows down metabolism in order to save energy. Eating regularly fuels your body making sure that it works at its peak by increasing its metabolic rate.

iv) Balances hormones

Our bodies have several hormones that play a crucial role in metabolism, hunger levels and weight loss. Some of those hormones are insulin and ghrelin.

When we eat regularly we ensure that we have a steady supply of insulin, which is needed to process sugar or glucose in our blood. When we stay for a long time without eating a lot of insulin is released when we eat. Large quantities of insulin in our bodies encourage the storage of fat and when the insulin spike crashes, we experience strong hunger pangs.

Ghrelin is also known as the hunger hormone. It is usually secreted when we go for a long time without eating. It slows down the rate at which your body utilizes stored fats and also increases appetite, which in turn increases, our urge to eat making us eat more than we actually need.

Small frequent meals are an important aspect of weight loss. Even more important is what you eat during those meals. In order to get maximum satisfaction each mini meal should contain a lean or low fat protein, fiber and very little healthy fat.

6. Eating raw fruits and vegetables

There are 3 reasons why raw food diets work.

i. Raw food is full of enzymes and enzymes control everything in your body. They help us to digest and break down the food we eat, and when we get good nutrients from the food we are less likely to over eat.

ii.An alkaline diet helps to remove acid wastes, or toxins from the body. This is because many of the acid toxins are encapsulated in your body fat. As the toxins are released your body also releases excess body fat. Losing weight in this case may be as simple as balancing the body Ph.

iii.Raw foods are not calorie dense foods, which means you can eat to your filling and take in far less calories than if the food would have been cooked. Raw foods are also full of fiber that will promote regular bowel movements.

How to include raw food in your diet

For most people, switching to raw food would be a big change. However to experience real and effective weight loss, you do not have to eat 100% raw food, or do anything that does not feel comfortable to you. The most important thing is to eatmore raw food than you are used to. For starters anything is an improvement as you are moving away from food that is processed towards more natural food.

The more you eat raw food as compared to cooked and processed food, the more toxins and excess weight you lose. It is important to note that making huge changes from an unIntuitive nutritional therapy to 100% raw diet is extremely demanding. It is beneficial to make your transition gently.

You can start with baby steps. This means that you can start eating fruits for lunch, having salads with all cooked meals and choosing all raw snacks.

7. Be more active

Our biggest health hazard is all the time you spend sitting. For many people, daily routines dictate how much time we spend while seated.

You can also split your activity into several short periods instead of completing it in one go. Choose activities that you will enjoy and can fit into your schedule. It may take time to incorporate more activity into your life. Do not be discouraged you miss a day or two; keep trying until you make it a regular part of your life. You will eventually realize that being physically active and fit makes you feel good.

Seek support from family and friends and join other people who are trying to be physically active. Many of physical activities can be social, allowing you to spend time with family and friends.

Being active does not only involve exercise, it simply means getting off the couch or chair and doing something. For example doing chores, walking the dog, walking to the grocery store or even playing with your children.

When at work you can take stairs instead of the lift or take a walk during your tea or lunch break.

8. Prepare and cook your own food

When it comes to weight loss, you should not depend on others to nourish you. Food that is not prepared in your home is not in your control. Most times, it will be loaded with salt and fat. The only solution is to cook your own food.

Cook larger meals so that you have leftovers to eat for the days ahead. Shop for fresh and organic food in the local market.Fresh produce is always better than processed and frozen varieties.

Benefits of preparing your own food

i) Helps you to save money

Instead of spending hundreds of dollars a month eating out, make your own budget and lose weight by eating at home more often. The money that you use to eat out once can be enough to buy groceries for 3-4 meals.

ii) Portion control

People tend to eat more when they are served larger portions. This makes it a challenge when you are eating out because the portions in many restaurants exceed what is recommended. Home cooking makes you control the portions, which limits calories that you consume hence you lose weight.

iii) Fat Content

The problem with processed foods and meals prepared at restaurants is that it is hard to know exactly how much fat they contain. A high fat content impacts weight because 1 gram of fat has 9 calories, compared to only 4 calories in 1 gram of carbohydrates and proteins. Preparing your own meals lets you control the amount of fat you add in your food. In addition you can choose to use low-fat cooking methods like steaming and you can also substitute fats with healthier choices. A good example preparing lean ground beef patty broiled at home contains only 145 calories, compared to 254 calories found in a fast food hamburger patty.

iv) Food Choices

Eating out limited choices of what you can order. Even though some restaurants allow you to make healthy substitutions, the ultimate opportunity for food choice is only found at home. Increasing the amount of vegetables, fruits, beans and whole grains significantly increases nutrients, and decreases calories and supports efforts to lose weight.

9. Use healthy substitutes for unhealthy food

Staying healthy means having a wide variety of healthy alternatives to choose from. Healthy alternatives instead of junk food can help in improve your health.

Unfortunately, with junk food being sold everywhere it becomes difficult to make healthy choices. Unhealthy food that is high in sugar, sodium and fat are more readily available and more convenient than their healthy counterparts. However for someone who is dedicated to improving his/her health and losing weight there are several substitutions they can make.

10. Get more rest

As wild as the idea sounds medical evidence suggests some links between sleep and weight. According to researchers how much you sleep and quite possibility the quality of your sleep may be linked to your appetite.

Although doctors have known for a long time that many hormones are affected by sleep, it wasn't until recently that appetite entered the picture. Research on the hormones leptin and ghrelin are what brought it into focus. According to doctors,both hormones can influence our appetite and also production of both may be influenced by how much or how little we sleep.

Leptin and ghrelin work in a kind of "checks and balances" system to control feelings of hunger and fullness. Ghrelin, which is produced in the gastrointestinal tract, stimulates appetite, while leptin, which is produced in fat cells, sends a signal to the brain when you are satisfied.

The result is that when you do not get enough sleep, leptin levels fall, which means you don't feel as satisfied after you eat. Lack of sleep also causes ghrelin levels to rise, which means your appetite is stimulated, so you have an urge to eat more food.

When you combine the two hormones you can set the stage for overeating, which in turn may lead to weight gain.

Getting enough sleep will balance your body's hormones and reduce urges to overeat. It also gives you less time to engage in activities that make you over indulge.

11. Exercise

Exercise is an effective way to improve both your physical and mental health. Besides reducing your risk of serious health problems, some regular exercise can help relieve depression and anxiety, increase energy and mood and relieve stress.

Benefits of exercise

Exercise is not only about aerobic capacity and muscle mass. Although exercise can improve your health and your body, trim your waistline, improve your sex life and even add years to your life, it is not what most people need to motivate them to stay active. People who exercise regularly tend to do so because it gives them a tremendous sense of well-being. You feel more energetic throughout the day, sleep better at night, have sharper memories, and feel relaxed and positive about themselves and their lives. And it does not take hours pumping weights in a gym or running mile after mile to achieve these results.

By focusing on activities that you enjoy and easily design a moderate regular exercise routine to suit your needs, you will experience the health benefits of exercise and improve your own life by:

i. Easing stress and anxiety.

Twenty minutes bike ride will not sweep all the problems of life, but regular exercise helps you to handle anxiety and reduce stress.

iii. Sharpening brainpower.

Endorphins make you feel better also help you to concentrate and feel mentally sharp for tasks at hand. Exercise stimulates the growth of new brain cells and helps prevent age-related decline.

iv. Improving self-esteem.

Regular activity is an investment in your mind, body, and soul. When you make it a habit, it can increase your sense of self-worth and make you feel strong and powerful.

v. Boosting energy.

Exercise increases your heart rate giving you more energy to get up and go. You should start off with just a few minutes of activity a day, and increase the intensity of your workout as you feel more energized.

Obstacles to exercise

Despite all the advantages of exercise, many of us still think of exercise as an optional chore, something that we don't have time for, or something that we do not have to do everyday.

Conquering the excuses that we give ourselves for not exercising requires separating fact from fiction.

i. Lack of time

Short low-impact intervals of exercise can be very beneficial to your health. If you have time for a 15-minute workout, your body will thank you in many ways. In the end a little exercise is much better than none.

ii. Lack of motivation

Exercise does not only mean going to the gym for an intense workout. You can work out by simply doing things that you enjoy. You don't have to push yourself to the limit to get results. You can build your strength and fitness by simply walking, swimming, even playing golf or cleaning the house.

iii. Fatigue

Regular exercise is a great way to combat fatigue. If you are feeling tired, a brisk walk or dancing to your favorite music will make you feel much better

iv. Age

Physical activity is important no matter what age you are. Exercise is a proven treatment for many diseases such as diabetes and arthritis. Very few health or weight problems make exercise out of the question, so talk to your doctor about a safe routine for you.

v. Level of fitness

As mentioned before workouts do not have to be high intensity. You can always start small and increase your intensity at the rate you are most comfortable with.

vi. Boredom

Running on a treadmill for 60 minutes may not be every ones cup of tea. In any case not all practice must be exhausting; practically every one can discover a physical action they like. Purported "exergames" that are played standing up and moving around can burn in any event the same amount calories as strolling on a treadmill and maybe considerably more. This will help you lose weight but in a fun way.

12. Keep a food journal

Keeping a food journal could make you more successful in losing weight and keeping it off. In fact, people who keep a food diary lose twice as much as those who do not.

Keeping a food diary increases your awareness of what you eat, how much of it that you consume, and why you are eating. This ensures that you eat the right food, at the right time.

A food diary will also help you to identify areas where you can make changes that will help you lose weight.

Food diaries can help reveal patterns of overeating. They can also show you the triggers to avoid. For example you can know that not eating enough during the day will trigger overeating at night, or drinking alcohol triggers overeating.

In some cases, the fact that you have to record every bite helps deter you from overeating you will often reconsider eating something because you do not want to write it down.

Living healthy is not only about weight loss; it is about moving your body and nourishing it with good things for health and longevity.

Making lifestyle changes is a medley of weight loss guidelines that will always stay genuine irrespective of which program you pick. Still there are some facts that will remain consistent when it comes to weight loss and they are:

• 3500 calories is equivalent to one pound (.05 kilogram) of fat.

• You must burn 500 to 1,000 calories more than what you ingest each day in order to drop 1 to 2 pounds a week.

• Working out is the fundamental to burning extra calories.

• Walking is one of the best sources of aerobic workouts to burn body fat

• Take the steps instead of the elevator, and park far away from the building in order to increase number of daily steps.

• You should aim for 10,000 steps of walking every day.

• Breakfast is the most vital meal of the day when trying to lose weight

13. Think positive

Positive views play a major role in your weight loss efforts. Continuous negative thoughts can lead to self-defeating behaviors such as deviating from your diet, binging and missing your exercise routine. Positive thoughts, on the other hand, can increase your drive and energy level.

Positive Thinking and Weight Loss

Positive thoughts are inspiring. A negative stance can set processes in action that makes losing weight tough, if not unmanageable. Criticizing yourself every time you have the wrong foods, always concentrating on what you cannot eat and approaching your exercise schedule with anxiety are all ways that unhelpful thought patterns can disrupt your weight loss efforts.

When you hold a negative image of yourself, you deprive yourself of much-needed energy. When feeling helpless, miserable or unmotivated, it becomes easy to avoid your daily workout or consume a bag of potato chips to help you feel better. Nevertheless, tuning into how you feel, accepting those feelings and altering those thoughts into something more positive can truly help you to reach your weight loss goals sooner.

How to increase positive thinking

Positive thinking is only successful if it is in line with your genuine feelings. If you honestly feel down about your body weight, telling yourself that all is fine will repeatedly create internal conflict.

The trick is to tap into those feelings that are true for you. For example, you can keep a daily journal where you write down your negative feelings and thoughts. If you are lacking in drive or just can't overcome your own food cravings, write those reflections down. When you accept the darker emotions, they often tend to have less authority over you.

It is critical to make a deliberate effort to change your thoughts. It could be right that you often cannot overcome your food cravings or stick to your diet and there are times when you are able to be resilient, then, concentrate on those moments and applaud yourself for the triumphs. Paying attention to the positive things will help to build a greater self-esteem and enthusiasm to continue with your weight loss efforts.

Setting Manageable Goals

A bad attitude can occur during dieting if you set difficult objectives for yourself. Trying to live on a tremendously low-calorie diet or setting your weekly weight loss target at an unachievable figure often sets you up for disaster.

In order to increase weight loss success, set attainable goals. Dropping one or two pounds per week is a practical goal and can generally be realized without severe measures.

You should weigh yourself weekly and each week you attain your goal, celebrate your success. This will maintain positive thinking. Before long, you will find that your motivation and energy have increased, and the pounds are dropping.

14. Meditate

Meditation, when performed accurately, indeed can increase your body's ability to shed pounds. When you force yourself to and concentrate on a peaceful object or mantra for a prolonged period of time, can reduce stress, lower blood pressure, and encourage a sense of inner focus.

The focus on breathing, posture, and the encouragement to probe into your own soul is surely mind opening and exciting. The body will appreciate this abrupt flow of serenity that runs within it after being relentlessly abused from the anxieties of day-to-day life.

Because of the stress relief and relaxation effects that meditation offers, it can be rather valuable to emotional eaters. Emotional eaters are those who tend to eat not so much out of hunger, but rather out of a need to fill some kind of emptiness. That "vacuum" may occur due to an a stressful day at work, an fight with a spouse, disappointment in a child, fear of the future, or anything that triggers you to feel an onset of formidable emotions.

Contrary to what many think, emotional eating can also be triggered by extreme happiness as well. The body does not have the ability in most cases to differentiate between good or bad stressors, and it will respond in the same manner to both in some ways. Consequently, even modest daily happenings can cause overeating, particularly if you are not aware that you eat food as a response to these situations and you do so without ever identifying the problem.

Meditation can be used to create balance and harmony in the mind, body, and soul, and it can become an alternative for the food that was previously used in its place.

Meditation starts with a "stillness" of the mind. Certainly, many people discover that it best to sit in a discreet room with candles lit and no disturbances around them while meditating, though this is not always possible in everyday situations.

You may meditate at the workplace, during lessons, or even during an intense fight. All that is required is that you master being in control of your thoughts. You must discover how to block disturbances. This is simpler said than done, but once it is attained, you will find yourself becoming more focused in every part of your life.

Preferably, you will begin in a quiet room with a relaxing CD softly playing in the background. Make sure that the CD is instrumental only or a "nature sounds" selection, as words can place pictures in your mind that should not be there as you try to clear your thoughts. Subsequently, sit either with legs straight in front of you on the floor or with them crossed, and close your eyes. Now, in order to totally clear your mind, concentrate on a serene, inorganic object or picture.

For example you can think of a beautiful sunset or a tree whose branches are swaying in the wind.If nature does not do it for you,imagine yourself living a better life. Continue to do so for as long as you wish, being cautious to elude all negative thoughts and qualms

The effects of meditation cannot be ignored. Used for centuries to help people concentrate on devotion, prayer, and spiritual strength, it is now being noticed for its weight loss benefits. The stress hormone cortisol is thought to decrease the body's ability to combat fat.

Consequently, allowing yourself a few moments a day to release this hormone can certainly lead to a weight loss increase. In women particularly, cortisol can be, not only harmful to weight loss goals, but also hazardous for the entire body. Taking a few moments a day to meditate on something rather than the hustle and bustle of life, and combine that with your diet and weight loss routine will ensure that you have a successful weight loss journey

CHAPTER NINE

Key to Optimal Health

Optimal health means more than the absence of pain, sickness and disease. As important as it is to be physical healthy it is equally important to be mentally, emotionally and spiritually healthy as well. Optimal health, therefore, in context of what is being written here, is a balance of physical, mental, emotional, and spiritual aspects of health. Let us take a look at each of these aspects, beginning with physical health.

Physical Health

So much has been written about the subject of physical health in the categories of health and wellness, diet and weight loss, fitness and bodybuilding etc. In this article I will primarily deal with physical health in its internal aspect which includes building a healthy immune system, detoxifying the body, healthy and quick elimination, and nourishing the cells with proper nutrition. Aging itself can be slowed down by keeping the internal aspect of our physical health up to par. Wouldn't you love to have a healthy, youthful, energetic, strong, lean body which is free of disease, sickness and pain well into adulthood beyond the age of 40? It all narrows down to what type of food we put into our bodies - either food filled with toxins and poisons, or healthy, living, vital food.

Food is intended to furnish the body with all the live elements needed for the regeneration of its cells and tissues. If the body fails to be healthy, the lack or deficiency of regenerative elements in the food is the cause of, and the responsibility for, whatever ailment, sickness or disease overtakes it. Our bodies seek homeostasis, equilibrium, balance. This equals health. When given the right building blocks to work with, the body maintains itself in health.

These building blocks can be found in whole, unbleached, organic grains, rice (wild rice, brown rice etc.), beans, fruits, vegetables, nuts, various seeds and herbs etc. Large portions of these building blocks can be found in the "super-food" family in such foods as Spirulina and Barley Grass. (A super-food is extremely rich in a large variety of vitamins, minerals, trace minerals and amino acids, and can be assimilated by our bodies very easily. Spirulina is a complete protein and is known to be very healthy.) Look in your local health food store for super green foods in powdered form. I personally sometimes use Garden of Life Perfect Food Super Green Formula.

Super-foods are known to:

- Deter Aging
- Massively Boost Your Immune System
- Aid Weight Loss
- Lower Your Cholesterol
- Radically Improve Your Energy
- Enhance Your Mental & Emotional Well-being
- Boost Your Libido
- Alkalize Your System

- Protect against Toxins and Pollutants

- Beautify Your Skin

- Cleanse and Fortify Your Blood

- Nourish and Revitalize your Systems

Fight and Protect against numerous diseases including Diabetes, Hypertension, Heart Disease, Stroke, Cancer, Arthritis, Cataracts, Osteoporosis, Acne, Obesity, High cholesterol, Age-Related Blindness...And Much More!

"By taking just a bit of a super-food (in capsule or powered drink form) as a supplement to your diet, you will find many wonderful things happen to your body. Essentially, the nourishment will give your body the needed resources to rebuild any broken or damaged parts and improve your body's chances of returning to homeostasis. Testimonies of its power range from improved eyesight, to relief from back pain, to better scores in sports by world champion competitive athletes. Generally, one will experience feelings of increased energy and vitality; reduction and alleviation of stress, anxiety and depression; relief from the discomforting symptoms of fatigue, hypoglycemia, some allergies, poor digestion and sluggishness; and improved memory and mental clarity. People also experience elimination of mood swings, toxin elimination, better sleep, reduced cravings for food and sweets, lower blood pressure and many other health benefits. Then there are many specialized health problems which have disappeared as people's bodies receive adequate nutrition through super-foods. Prostate problems have been normalized, as well as triglycerides, arthritis and diabetes, and many other severe and degenerative diseases. Basically, any and every disease will be fought off by your body, if it has the right tools to fight with. Super-foods give it the right tools. You just need to try it for thirty days and see what it may do for you. I recommend taking a product that includes several kinds of super foods, as they work together in a synergy that can have a profound effect on your health and vitality. If your body needs detoxifying first, you may experience a bit of a "tissue cleansing" during the first few days or weeks of taking the super-food as your body cleanses itself."

Basically if we put the wrong food (and drink) into our body it weakens the immune system and opens the door for us to be susceptible to health problems of whatever sort (whether it be frequents colds and sicknesses, flues, aches and pains, sores and ulcers, weakness, sluggishness, high blood pressure, high cholesterol, arthritis, heart problems, diabetes, cancer or psychological disorders such as malaise, apathy or memory problems etc., etc., etc.) Looking on the bright side a healthy immune system that is not swamped with toxins can fight off diseases successfully!

It is preferable to never be unhealthy to begin with and to eat nothing but healthy food from day one. Unfortunately it is not this way. Many have been conditioned to eat unhealthy, fattening, artery clogging foods from childhood to the grave. Many of us think it is a normal part of the aging process to start getting weaker, fatter, having more pain etc. after age 30 and onward. In many cases (definitely not all) premature aging and bodily weakening is the result of years of poor eating habits from childhood to adulthood. Due to many years of wrong eating habits it may be best to detoxify.

In the process of nourishing our cells with foods high in fiber such as vegetables, fruits, super-foods, and whole grains our body naturally detoxifies itself in the process, which in turn strengthens our immune system and slows, or in some cases, reverses the aging process. The key to optimal health as far as the physical aspect of our health goes, is to:

Eat plenty of Grains, vegetables, fruits, nuts, super-foods, herbs, being sure to get plenty of exercise, pure water and clean air, excreting waste from the intestines quickly (which is a byproduct of eating plenty of fruits, fiber and vegetables). There are also natural supplements you can take such as Vitamin C, vitamins and minerals, and various antioxidants unless you are getting plenty of these from your regular diet.

Mental and Emotional Health

Mental and emotional health are so closely related it is hard to separate the two. Having a healthy mind is not limited to having a keen intellect and an excellent memory. Someone can excel at this level of mental health but still be an emotional wreck, not to mention being spiritually ignorant at the same time.

Negative mental attitudes or emotions can have a direct effect on our physical health even if we are eating healthy food. Emotional traumas, anger, rage, hate, stress etc., when persisted in day in and day out, weaken the immune system and manifest in ill physical health. A negative mind, over time, often erases all the good that healthy food does for us.

Some forms of sickness, disease, and illness, as well as bad habits like smoking, drinking, drugs etc., are often external symptoms of something deeper. They are effects of a deeper cause. And until that cause is addressed and healed the symptoms will keep coming back like fruit on a tree whether in the form of ill health, disease, anxiety, bad habits of one sort or another, or in the worse case scenario cancer. Luckily there are warning signs when all is not well within.

The subconscious part of our mind is the storehouse of our emotions and memories and it is here where we need healing as far as our mental and emotional life are concerned. Sometimes negative or uneasy dreams (some of which originate from the sub conscious) are manifestations of our own fears and internal wounds. Some dreams are also messages, clothed with images we can comprehend, from our highest level of mind - the super conscious level - warning us when we are making wrong decisions, or heading in a wrong direction. In those rare cases where we are susceptible to the healing energies of the super conscious level of mind we can experience internal healing quicker than we ever imagined. More about this in a minute when I get to the spiritual aspect of health.

Along with a Intuitive nutritional therapy it is important to think positive thoughts and maintain a positive attitude, avoiding anger and bitterness towards others. But, thinking positive thoughts and making an effort to be happy, loving, and optimistic, are only part of what is involved when it comes to the healing of our emotional life. We can only go so far by exercising will power alone, as important as it is to use our own efforts when attempting to make a change in our emotional life for the better. All our ethical standards, our rules and regulations for leading an acceptable moral life, all our positive thinking formula are a means to an end, the end being the opening and revelation of the spiritual aspect or our mind - the super conscious level of mind. This brings me to the last category of health, the spiritual category.

Spiritual Health

I have written about this subject elsewhere and will be repeating some of the information here. Keep in mind when reading this that being spiritual is not to be confused with being religious. Someone who is religious can be operating from a physical, emotional, and mental level only, but be void as far as being spiritual goes. A pseudo religious life (not to be confused with a genuine religious life) that is lived in pride, elitism, self righteousness and egoism is completely opposite of spiritual life. In context of this article being spiritual means living your life from the level of your super conscious mind, and living a harmonious life naturally from that level. This is easier said than done because our pride and ego often get in the way and cause us untold pain and suffering. But by living in harmony with the super-conscious level of our mind, and accessing the spiritual grace and energy which flow through (from God and Spirit) that same level of mind, our mental and emotional health, as well as our physical health, all fall into place and are balanced.

All our moral, ethical, religious or merely human efforts at trying to be a more loving, positive, optimistic person are a feeble way of (often unconsciously) aligning, or attempting to align, ourselves with that ever present flow of energy, light, grace, and Spirit permeating throughout all creation.

This ever present, but often unperceived and untapped, spiritual energy upholding all creation is the source of a truly happy life even when we find ourselves in the midst of negative external circumstances. It is the ultimate key to optimal health. Some call this ever present energy cosmic consciousness, super-consciousness, Christ consciousness, God, Spirit, a Higher Power etc. Some people personalize it and clothe it with a human form and then worship the person it manifests through. Ancient writings say the heavens and earth were made by the word of God and by the breath of his mouth. This is a human way of trying to accommodate a spiritual truth to the limited understanding of the human brain, using analogies, parables, particular genders, and concepts that can be understood by the rational brain. This often results in misunderstandings and even war and bloodshed in the name of religion.

The naked truth is intuitively perceived by the higher aspect of human consciousness called super consciousness. And it is this level of consciousness (Christ consciousness) that wells up from within to "save," change, deliver, and heal us when the thick layer of ego, all the emotional blockages, wounded memories, and wrong thinking, are thinned out enough by our own efforts at self improvement. This is the truth of the "Messiah" or Savior figure often mentioned in ancient writings. Eventually we have to let go of our own strivings and let God take over.

Or, we can continue to resist the inner pull and instead live an unnatural life with the end result of disharmony on all levels physical, mental and emotional. (This is the truth about the so called wrath of God. It has nothing to do God or Spirit being angry at us. But it has everything to do with us bringing suffering upon ourselves by choosing to go our own way, not heeding the whispers and impressions of the super conscious mind either within ourselves, or speaking through dreams, visions, other people, or even through writing, art, and so on.)

Once we tap into the spiritual flow of grace then a truly changed person is the result, from the inside out. Children are closer to this level of being than adults who have been conditioned and brainwashed throughout life via peer pressure, upbringing, culture and so on. Humility is key, not pride and ego. Attaining to the spiritual level of healing consciousness is the end of all religions.

CONCLUSION

Health is your most valuable asset and it is ironic that many people tend only to appreciate how important health is when they fall ill or someone close to them is suffering from ill health. It is very important that you take care of your health and make sure that you are properly looked after. A lot of people fail to realize that if you do nothing in regard to your health now, you will likely end up with ill health down the track and then trying to seek some help might be too late as you may have already done irreparable damage to yourself. Following are some helpful tips that might help you to look after your health:

It is important to get regular health check ups under the supervision of a registered physician or qualified doctor. Regular check ups help you to keep an eye on your general health and fitness. They also help to rectify or treat any medical conditions or diseases at its initial stages. Always practice safe sex techniques and make sure you use condoms during sexual activities. Cut down on your daily alcohol intake and stick to the recommended guidelines for the daily drinking. Be careful with the amount of caffeine you take in a day as excessive caffeine may interfere with your sleep. Another good thing you can do for the sake of your health is quit smoking if you are a smoker. The gases that you inhale when you smoke a cigarette are very bad for your health and may lead to cancer and other heart related problems.

You need to include a balanced diet in your regular daily routine. Raw vegetables and fresh fruits are a great source of vital nutrients and will play a key role in keeping you healthy and fit. They provide you with all the vitamins, minerals, antioxidants and fiber that your body needs to stay healthy and active. Include organic lean meats, complex carbohydrates, and healthy fats in your diet on a daily basis. Avoid excessive sugar and fatty foods from junk food sources. Drink adequate liquids especially water. Water is a great cleansing agent and it helps carry harmful toxins out of your body. It also regulates the temperature of your body and keeps you hydrated and functioning optimally. It is generally recommended to take around 8-10 glasses of good clean water every day.

It is also important that you exercise regularly. Regular exercise not only keeps you physically healthy and fit; it also helps you mentally and will help keep you smart and confident. A regular exercise detoxifies your body naturally through sweating and as a result is great for body detoxification. Try to exercise for 30-45 minutes daily. Among different exercises, you can practice Pilates or yoga if this suits you, and basic movements like chin ups, push ups, deadlifts, lunges, front and side planks, and squats will give you all the muscle tone and strength you need and keep your body functional and healthy.